OXFORD HIGHER SPECIALTY TRAINING

Viva Training in ENT

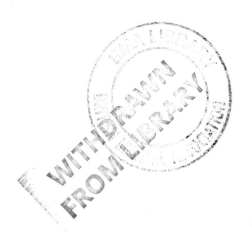

OXFORD HIGHER SPECIALTY TRAINING

Viva Training in ENT

Preparation for the FRCS (ORL-HNS)

EDITED BY

Declan Costello
Consultant ENT Surgeon, Queen Elizabeth Hospital, Birmingham

Stuart Winter
Consultant ENT Surgeon, Head and Neck Surgeon, Oxford University Hospitals

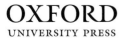

OXFORD
UNIVERSITY PRESS

OXFORD
UNIVERSITY PRESS

Great Clarendon Street, Oxford, OX2 6DP,
United Kingdom

Oxford University Press is a department of the University of Oxford.
It furthers the University's objective of excellence in research, scholarship,
and education by publishing worldwide. Oxford is a registered trade mark of
Oxford University Press in the UK and in certain other countries

British Library Cataloguing in Publication Data

Data available

ISBN 978–0–19–965950–0 (pbk.)

Printed in Great Britain by
CPI Group (UK) Ltd, Croydon, CR0 4YY

Contents

Contributors

Rogan Corbridge *Chapter 2*
Consultant ENT Surgeon, Royal Berkshire Hospital, Reading

Declan Costello *Editor, Chapter 5, Chapter 6*
Consultant ENT Surgeon, Queen Elizabeth Hospital, Birmingham

Alison Hunt *Chapter 1*
Specialist Registrar in ENT Surgery, John Radcliffe Hospital, Oxford

Michael Kuo *Chapter 4*
Consultant Paediatric ENT Surgeon, Birmingham Children's Hospital, Birmingham

Samuel MacKeith *Chapter 3*
ENT Specialist Registrar, Oxford Deanery, Oxford

Victoria Possamai *Chapter 4*
Specialist Registrar in ENT Surgery, West Midlands Rotation

James Ramsden *Chapter 3*
Consultant ENT Surgeon, Oxford University Hospitals, Oxford

Stuart Winter *Editor, Chapter 7*
Consultant ENT Surgeon, Head and Neck Surgeon, Oxford University Hospitals, Oxford

Abbreviations

AABR	automated auditory brainstem response
ABR	auditory brainstem response
AC	air conduction
ACE	angiotensin-converting enzyme
AN	acoustic neuroma
AOAE	automated oto-acoustic emission
AOM	acute otitis media
AP	action potential
AVM	arteriovenous malformations
b/w	black & white
BAHA	bone anchored hearing aid
BC	bone conduction
BCC	basal cell carcinoma
BKB	Bamford–Kowal–Bench
BMI	body mass index
BP	blood pressure
BPPV	benign paroxysmal positional vertigo
CAMP	compound muscle action potential
cANCA	cytoplasmic antineutrophil cytoplasmic antibody
CAT	combined approach tympanoplasty
CERA	cortical electrical response audiometry
CI	cochlear implant
CM	cochlear microphonic
CMV	cytomegalovirus
CN	cranial nerve
CN V	cranial nerve five (trigeminal nerve)
CNS	central nervous system
CPA	cerebellopontine angle
CPAP	continuous positive airways pressure
CRP	C-reactive protein
CSF	cerebrospinal fluid
CSOM	chronic suppurative otitis media
CT	computed tomography
CVA	cerebrovascular accident
CXR	chest X-ray
DR	dynamic range
DVLA	Driver and Vehicle Licensing Authority
DXT	radiotherapy
EAC	external auditory canal
ECA	external carotid artery
ECG	electrocardiogram
ECMO	extra-corporeal membrane oxygenation
ECoG	electrocochleography
ELS	endolymphatic sac
EMG	electromyography
ENT	ear, nose, and throat
ESR	erythrocyte sedimentation rate

ET	endotracheal
ETD	Eustachian tube dysfunction
FBC	full blood count
FEES	Functional Endoscopic Evaluation of the Swallowing
FESS	functional endoscopic sinus surgery
FNA	fine needle aspiration
FNAC	fine needle aspiration cytology
FNE	flexible nasendoscopy
FRCS	Fellow of the Royal College of Surgeons
G+S	group and save
GA	general anaesthetic
GCS	Glasgow Coma Score
GJB2	gap junction beta 2
GMC	General Medical Council
HHT	haemorrhagic telangiectasia
HIB	*Haemophilus influenza* type B
HME	heat and moisture exchanger
HPV	human papilloma virus
HR	heart rate
HVDT	health visitor distraction test
IAM	internal acoustic meatus
ICA	internal carotid artery
IJV	internal jugular vein
IMA	inferior meatal antrostomy
ISJ	incudostapedial joint
ITU	intensive care unit
JNA	juvenile nasal angiofibroma
KTP	potassium-titanyl phosphate
LA	local anaesthetic
LMN	lower motor neurone palsy
LN	lymph node
MDT	multi-disciplinary team
MRI	magnetic resonance imaging
NG	nasogastric
NGT	nasogastric tube
NHSP	Newborn Hearing Screening Programme
NICU	neonatal intensive care unit
NIHL	noise-induced hearing loss
NOHL	non-organic hearing loss
OAE	otoacoustic emission
OME	otitis media with effusion
OPD	outpatients department
OPG	orthopantomogram
OSA	obstructive sleep apnoea
PAN	polyarteritis nodosa
PCR	polymerase chain reaction
PDT	photodynamic therapy
PE	pharyngo-oesophageal
PEG	percutaneous endoscopic gastrostomy
PICU	paediatric intensive care unit

PNS	post-nasal space
PPI	proton pump inhibitor
PTA	pure tone audiogram
PTS	permanent threshold shift
RLN	recurrent laryngeal nerve
RND	radical neck dissection
RR	respiration rate
RRP	recurrent respiratory papillomatosis
SALT	speech and language therapy
SCBU	special care baby unit
SCC	squamous cell carcinoma
SCC	semicircular canal
SCM	sternocleidomastoid
SIADH	syndrome of inappropriate anti-diuretic hormone secretion
SLE	systemic lupus erythematosus
SM	submental
SNHL	sensorineural hearing loss
SP	summating potential
SPECT	single photo emission computed tomography
SPL	sound pressure level
TFT	thyroid function test
TM	tympanic membrane
TNM	tumour, nodes, metastasis
TTS	temporary threshold shifts
U&E	urea & electrolytes
UPSIT	University of Pennsylvania Smell Identification Test
URT	upper respiratory tract
URTI	upper respiratory tract infection
VC	vocal cord
VS	vestibular schwanomma

Introduction

This book has been written principally for candidates sitting the Intercollegiate FRCS (ORL-HNS) Section 2 examination. We have tried to replicate the format and style of questioning used in the examination.

The questions have been compiled by surgeons who have an understanding of what the examination requires and the depth of knowledge they anticipate is needed. We would like to thank everyone who has contributed their time so generously.

The style of the book was chosen to provide an idea of the answers needed, but clearly in a *viva voce* setting the delivery will depend on your personal approach.

In general terms, the purpose of the examination is to prepare 'safe' surgeons with a good working clinical knowledge of otolaryngology practice. It is unusual for examiners to try to trick the candidates into giving the wrong answer; they are keen to award marks, rather than find reasons to remove them.

The examiners wish to see candidates they can trust, and who they would consider to be good colleagues. You should approach the examination as you would approach your everyday clinical practice—when thinking of a differential diagnosis, mention the common conditions first; when speaking to a patient, be courteous and thoughtful.

Our feeling is that the examination, while having pre-set questions, remains a very fluid experience in which there is a great opportunity to influence the direction of questioning. While we hope this book gives you some idea of the breadth and depth of knowledge needed, it does not replace practising answering questions.

The chapters of the book are divided into the different sections of the examination. You will notice that the 'model answers' are given mostly in bullet point format; these will cover the main topics that should be mentioned, but your ability to translate these into a cogent well-reasoned verbal response is a matter of practise.

Although this book will present a useful adjunct to revision, there is no substitute for practising Viva technique—take every opportunity to practise your Viva technique with your peers, and seek assistance from consultant colleagues.

Psychological preparation for the examination is very important—it is critical to arrive at the examination in a calm, well-rested state of mind.

We hope you find the book stimulating and useful for the examination. Good luck.

Declan Costello
Stuart Winter

Notes on the format of the FRCS examination Section 2

Up-to-date examination regulations can be found at: http://www.intercollegiate.org.uk/

As of the time of printing, the examination is broken into the following sections (this information is taken from the Intercollegiate website):

1. Oral examination (4 × 30-minute orals)

- Otology including neuro-otology
- Head and neck surgery

- Paediatric otolaryngology
- Rhinology and facial plastics—(facial plastics will cover otoplasty, rhinoplasty, flap reconstruction, excision of facial lesions, suturing techniques, tissue handling, and assessment of patients undergoing cosmetic procedures).

Each Viva table has two examiners who will alternate asking questions. Each 30-minute Viva in this section will generally be divided into six themes, each of 5 minutes.

2. Clinical examination

- History taking and communication skills (20 minutes)
- Clinical short cases on the following domains (two 20-minute sessions):

Otology including neuro-otology, paediatric otolaryngology, head and neck surgery, and rhinology and facial plastics.

3. Practical examination in operative surgery (20-minute session)

This will involve temporal bone dissection and may include cadaveric head and neck specimens, and endoscopic examination of the cadaveric nose.

Pertinent to which, candidates should have a knowledge of:

- Basic sciences
- Clinical presentation and progression of disease processes
- Investigative procedures
- Management policy of disease processes
- Operative techniques, including reconstruction.

Chapter 1

Facial plastics/rhinology

Question 1

1.1 Describe the photograph shown in Figure 1.1.1.

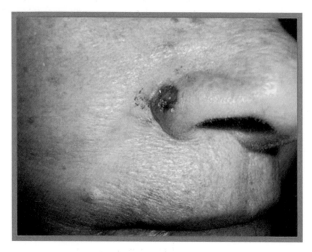

Figure 1.1.1

1.2 What types do you know and what is this one?

1.3 What are the surgical options for treatment?

1.4 What are the reconstructive options? Draw them.

1.5 Having excised the tumour, the histopathology shows that the excision margins are not clear. How might you ensure clear margins at time of primary surgery?

Answers to Question 1

1.1 Describe the photograph shown in Figure 1.1.1.

This photograph shows a lesion on the lateral aspect of the right ala. It is likely to represent a basal cell carcinoma (BCC) with characteristic features of raised pearly edge with telangiectasia and central ulceration.

History should focus on:

- Occupation
- Age
- Sun exposure
- Previous skin lesions.

Examination should focus on:

- Skin type (Fitzpatrick skin type, see Table 1.1.1)
- Examine other sun exposed areas
- Neck.

1	Very white, always burns, never tans
2	White, usually burns, tans minimally
3	White to olive, sometimes burns, tans
4	Brown, rarely burns, always tans
5	Dark brown rarely burns tans profusely
6	Black never burns, tans profusely

Table 1.1.1 Fitzpatrick Scale of Skin Types

BCC is the most common skin cancer, and is related to sun exposure. It is associated with mutation in *PTCH/P53* genes. In young patients with BCC one should consider Gorlin's syndrome. This rare syndrome is associated with BCC, odontogenic cysts, broad forehead, and palmar pits.

Histology of a typical BCC shows basaloid tumour cells arising from epidermis or follicles. It tends to spread locally, rather than to regional lymph nodes.

1.2 What types do you know and what is this one?

BCC is the most common cutaneous neoplasm, accounting for 60% of such growths.

- Nodular (classic BCC)
- Superficial (look like thin, erythematous, dry, scaly plaques)
- Morpheic (the most invasive type, this can look like a scar or plaque, usually around the nose)
- Pigmented (differential, here includes melanoma; it may be nodular or superficial).

1.3 What are the surgical options for treatment?

Excision with a 4-mm margin taking into account relaxed skin tension lines, facial subunits, and reconstruct using reconstructive ladder (see Table 1.1.2).

Secondary intention	Direct closure	Grafts (dead tissue, reliant on graft site for survival)	Local flaps Random vs. axial (based on named vessel)	Distal flaps regional	Free flaps	Prefabrication	Prosthetics

▶▶Increasing complexity

Table 1.1.2 The reconstructive ladder

1.4 What are the reconstructive options? Draw them.

Options include:

(i) Bilobed flap (interposition flap)—see Figure 1.1.2

(ii) Nasolabial flap (axial flap based on branches of facial artery)—see Figure 1.1.3

(iii) Advancement flap, but may need second stage procedure to create nasolabial crease.

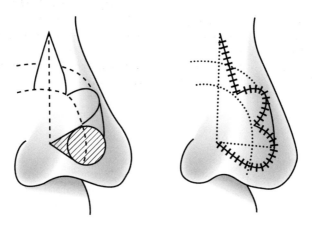

Figure 1.1.2 Bilobed flap.

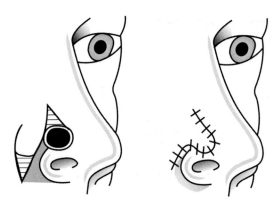

Figure 1.1.3 Nasolabial flap.

1.5 Having excised the tumour, the histopathology shows that the excision margins are not clear. How might you ensure clear margins at time of primary surgery?

Clear margins can be obtained by using frozen section or Moh's micrographic surgery. Moh's micrographic surgery is a technique used to gain total histological control.

The tumour is excised with standard margin, but with a 45-degree angle at its edge. The sample is then squashed and horizontally sectioned (in contrast to traditional vertical sectioning of a sample)

The sample is divided into colour-coded sections to make a tumour map, and the margins examined for tumour. If positive margins are found, the surgeon can repeat the exercise, removing more tissue until the margins are clear. This is the treatment of choice for high risk lesions. The cure rate, using this technique is >99% for new lesions and >95% for recurrent lesions.

Question 2

2.1 You are asked to see an 8-year-old girl with a grossly swollen, red, and tender left eyelid. How would you manage this patient?

2.2 Would you arrange imaging? What would you do?

2.3 Here is some imaging (see Figure 1.2.1). Tell me about it.

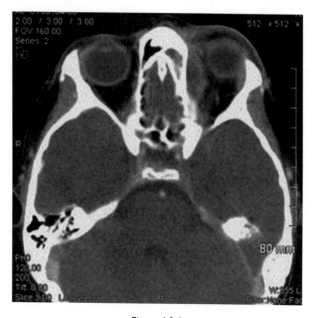

Figure 1.2.1

2.4 What classification do you know for this?

2.5 What are the signs in cavernous sinus thrombosis?

2.6 What surgery would you perform in a 6-year-old child with a sub-periosteal collection?

Answers to Question 2

2.1 You are asked to see an 8-year-old girl with a grossly swollen, red and tender left eyelid. How would you manage this patient?

This child has peri-orbital cellulitis.

History should focus on:

- Recent coryzal illness
- Any treatment already undertaken
- Pain on eye movement
- Duration of symptoms.

Examination should pay close attention to:

- Colour vision
- Visual acuity
- Afferent papillary light reflexes
- Range of movement
- Chemosis
- Proptosis
- Bilateral signs
- Reduced conscious level
- Examine the nose itself.

Arrange for regular eye observations, nasal examination, and organize an urgent ophthalmological opinion. Keep the child nil-by-mouth in case urgent surgical intervention is required.

In the absence of previous antibiotics, it would be reasonable to treat with intravenous antibiotics (co-amoxiclav), nasal steroid drops, and nasal decongestants.

2.2 Would you arrange imaging? What would you do?

This is an area for debate, and different papers in the literature will support either immediate computed tomography (CT) or CT in 24h if there is no improvement (see Box 1.2.1).

Box 1.2.1 Indications for immediate CT

These would include:

- Inability to assess vision
- Proptosis
- Ophthalmoplegia
- Bilateral oedema
- Deteriorating visual acuity
- Lack of improvement after 24h of administration of intravenous antibiotics
- 'Swinging' fevers not resolving within 36h
- Signs or symptoms of central nervous system (CNS) involvement.

Reproduced from Howe L, Jones NS. Guidelines for the management of periorbital cellulitis/abscess. *Clin Otolaryngol Allied Sci* 2004 Dec; **29**(6):725–8. Copyright 2004, with permission from John Wiley and Sons.

2.3 Here is some imaging (see Figure 1.2.1). Tell me about it.

This is an axial CT scan (with contrast) taken at the level of the orbits. It shows a subperiosteal abscess in the left orbit causing proptosis. Urgent intervention is now required.

2.4 What classification do you know for this?

Chandler's classification (see Box 1.2.2).

Box 1.2.2 **Chandler's classification**

I   Pre-septal
II   Post-septal without abscess
III Subperiosteal abscess
IV   Orbital abscess
V   Cavernous sinus thrombosis.

Reproduced from 'The pathogenesis of orbital complications in acute sinusitis', James R. Chandler, David J. Langenbrunner, Edward R. Stevens, *The Laryngoscope* **80**(9), 1414–28. Copyright 2009, with permission of John Wiley and Sons.

2.5 What are the signs in cavernous sinus thrombosis?

• Exophthalmos
• Paresis III/IV/VI
• Bilateral signs
• Reduced conscious level/cerebral irritation.

2.6 What surgery would you perform in a 6-year-old child with a sub-periosteal collection?

An **open approach** would be the more straightforward procedure, but would result in a scar and would necessitate the placement of a skin drain. A Lynch–Howarth incision (a curvilinear incision below the medial end of the eyebrow) is made. The dissection is deepened to the bone and the periosteum of the medial orbital wall is elevated posteriorly. The abscess will then be reached and drained. Comprehensive washout of the abscess cavity is performed with saline, and a corrugated drain is secured to the skin. It would be usual practice, under the same anaesthetic, to perform an antral washout (an intranasal puncture of the medial maxillary wall through the inferior meatus).

An **endoscopic approach** would entail uncinectomy, middle meatal antrostomy, and ethmoidectomy. The lamina papyracea is then elevated to drain the abscess. In a child of this age, the size of the nose can make endoscopic treatment difficult and a second procedure may be required 24–48h later if there is little improvement.

Question 3

A 36-year-old woman presents with left-sided watery rhinorrhoea for the last 9 months, getting progressively profuse. She has been trialled on a course of topical steroid spray without benefit. There is no history of facial trauma. A CT scan has been requested and is shown in Figure 1.3.1.

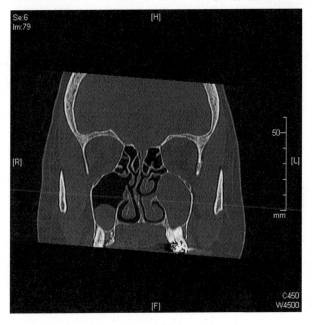

Figure 1.3.1

3.1 Describe the salient findings.

3.2 What tests are available to you to confirm it is cerebrospinal fluid (CSF)? Describe the Halo sign.

3.3 As part of her investigations she undergoes a CT spine cervical myelogram (see Figure 1.3.2). What does this demonstrate? What is the significance of this finding?

3.4 What are your treatment options?

3.5 What advice would you provide her with before surgery?

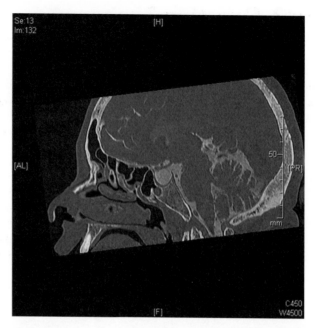

Figure 1.3.2

Answers to Question 3

3.1 Describe the salient findings.

Opacified left maxillary sinus and partial opacification of the right sinus. There is no evidence of bony destruction and these changes appear benign.

There is a bony defect of the floor of the left olfactory groove just posterior to the level of the crista galli.

3.2 What tests are available to you to confirm it is cerebrospinal fluid (CSF)? Describe the Halo sign.

Historically, the diagnosis was aided by the determining the presence of glucose and protein. A CSF leak existed when the glucose content exceeds 0.4g/l and the protein content is between 1 and 2g/l. However, the contamination of blood or other secretions often give a false positive.

The halo sign (or ring sign)—see Figure 1.3.3. Put some of the fluid onto a tissue. If there is CSF mixed with the blood, it will move by capillary action further away from the centre than the blood will.

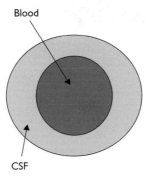

Figure 1.3.3 The halo sign.

The gold standard is to confirm that the fluid contains beta-2-transferrin.

3.3 As part of her investigations she undergoes a CT spine cervical myelogram (see Figure 1.3.2). What does this demonstrate? What is the significance of this finding?

There is significant enlargement of the pituitary fossa, which is almost completely empty. This appearance raises a suspicion of long-standing raised intracranial pressure (benign intracranial hypertension, BIH).

3.4 What are your treatment options?

While most cases of CSF leakage occurring after blunt trauma or skull base surgery resolve conservatively, this lady has had a prolonged leak.

Conservative measures include bed rest, elevation of the head, stool softeners, and the avoidance of straining. Lumbar drains or daily spinal CSF drainage have been utilized to lower the pressure.

Given the duration of this lady's symptoms, it is likely that she will require surgery to repair the defect. Given the possibility of raised intracranial pressure then discussion with a neurosurgeon and consideration of a peri-operative lumbar drain should be considered.

There are various surgical techniques described for repair of a skull base defect. The preferred option for this lady would be to utilize and endo-nasal technique. Intracranial and extracranial repairs are possible.

Surgical techniques include the use of overlay or underlay grafts. Most surgeons use local tissues to layer the repair or fat to plug it. Fibrin glue is frequently used to support the repair.

3.5 What advice would you provide her with before surgery?

- She needs to be warned about the symptoms of meningitis
- Prophylactic antibiotics still remain controversial.

Question 4

4.1 A 65-year-old lady presents to accident and emergency with a brisk epistaxis. How would you manage this lady?

4.2 How does silver nitrate cautery work?

4.3 This lady is admitted, but continues to bleed intermittently over several days despite repeat nasal packs and posterior packing. What are the options?

4.4 You arrange for a sphenopalatine artery ligation and anterior ethmoidal artery ligation. How would you perform this and what landmarks would you use?

Answers to Question 4

4.1 A 65-year-old lady presents to accident and emergency with a brisk epistaxis. How would you manage this lady?

Immediate management

- Control of the airway and breathing
- *Circulation*—adequate venous access (at the same time taking samples for full blood count (FBC), clotting, and a group and save).

Emergency measures

- Local pressure
- Ice packs are applied.

Brief history

Focus on:
- Anticoagulation/aspirin/clopidogrel
- Hypertension
- Any other significant medical history, including liver disease
- Recent nasal trauma/surgery
- Was the bleeding initially anterior or posterior; one side or both.

If the bleeding site is visible anteriorly cautery should be attempted under local anaesthetic. If this is unsuccessful, one should proceed to nasal packing. In the event of failure to control the bleeding with anterior nasal packs, posterior packs should be inserted.

4.2 How does silver nitrate cautery work?

Nitric acid is generated when $AgNO_3$ is mixed with H_2O, which creates chemical burn.

4.3 This lady is admitted, but continues to bleed intermittently over several days, despite repeat nasal packs and posterior packing. What are the options?

- *Surgery*—sphenopalatine artery ligation +/− anterior ethmoidal artery ligation
- Septoplasty if deviated septum
- External carotid artery ligation.

Embolization is also possible, but is reserved for resistant cases, where surgery contraindicated. Vessels greater than 2mm can be embolized, but carries significant risk of cerebrovascular accident (CVA)/dissection of vessels. This would need to be done in a specialist unit as these facilities are not always available locally.

4.4 You arrange for a sphenopalatine artery ligation and anterior ethmoidal artery ligation. How would you perform this and what landmarks would you use?

Anterior ethmoidal artery ligation

Lynch-Howarth incision down to bone, lifting periosteum and finding the lacrimal sac. The anterior ethmoidal artery is 24mm posterior to the anterior lacrimal crest, in the line of the fronto-ethmoidal suture. The posterior ethmoidal artery lies 12mm behind this. The optic nerve is 6mm behind this, but this distance varies between individuals and can be much closer. The artery may be diathermized, clipped, or both.

Sphenopalatine artery ligation

- Prepare the nose with lignocaine and adrenaline (one could also use Moffats—1ml of 1/1000 adrenaline, 2ml of 10% cocaine, 2ml of 8.4% sodium bicarbonate), prepared as for functional endoscopic sinus surgery (FESS), with patient head up, supine
- A mucoperiosteal flap is raised on the lateral nasal wall. The starting point for this flap is a vertical incision made approximately 1cm anterior to the posterior end of the middle turbinate, making an upper and lower incision with the Freer's to aid elevation
- The artery/branches of the artery can be seen just behind a bony spur, the crista ethmoidalis, which may need curette removal
- A ball seeker is useful to define the vessel, which may be diathermized, clipped, or both
- Having controlled the main vessel, it is imperative to examine for smaller additional branches and control them as well
- Avoid monopolar diathermy in view of the risk of optic nerve damage (it is just 10–13mm away), as arcing can occur
- Replace the flap and insert a small absorbable dressing to keep the flap in place. Formal packing is rarely required.

Question 5

5.1 What is hereditary haemorrhagic telangiectasia (HHT)?

5.2 What is the underlying pathology in HHT?

5.3 If you suspected HHT, what tests would you request and why?

5.4 How would you manage this patient?

Answers to Question 5

5.1 What is hereditary haemorrhagic telangiectasia (HHT)?

Also known as Osler–Rendu–Weber disease, it is characterized by recurrent epistaxis, telangiectasia, and arteriovenous malformations (AVM), which can occur in the brain, liver, or lung.

Easily visible telangiectasia typically occur in the nasal cavity, tongue, and on the lips.

5.2 What is the underlying pathology in HHT?

It is inherited in an autosomal dominant pattern, with a defect in the TGF β1 receptor gene, causing defect in contractile elements of blood vessels and abnormal angiogenesis resulting in telangiectasia and AVMs.

5.3 If you suspected HHT, what tests would you request and why?

CT of the chest, abdomen, and brain, as occult vascular malformations can be found here. The presence of three or more of the Curaçao criteria denote 'definite HHT':
- Spontaneous recurrent epistaxis
- Multiple telangiectasias in lung, liver, or brain
- Proven visceral AVMs
- First-degree family member with HHT.

If two of these criteria are met, the patient is said to have 'probable HHT'.

5.4 How would you manage this patient?

Conservative

- Iron supplementation
- Recurrent blood transfusion
- Absorbable packs
- Oestrogen creams
- Tranexamic acid
- Nasal obturators (occludes the nasal cavity).

Surgical

- *Cautery/LASER*—typically, the potassium-titanyl phosphate (KTP) laser is used to ablate the telangiectatic vessels
- Septodermoplasty (Saunders' procedure—skin graft to septum)
- Young's procedure (originally described 1967 for atrophic rhinitis)—a circumferential incision is made in the nasal mucosa 1cm inside the alar rim. The elevated mucosa is sutured together to close the nostril.

Question 6

A 23-year-old male presents with a life-long history of unilateral nasal discharge, mucoid, not bloody, and with no pus. It is constant and he is fed up with it. There is associated nasal blockage. He has come seeking your advice having tried a range of nasal sprays, to no avail.

6.1 What is your differential diagnosis?

6.2 CT scanning shows the following (see Figure 1.6.1). Tell me about this image.

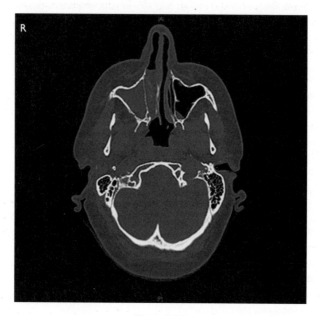

Figure 1.6.1

6.3 How would you manage this patient?

6.4 Do you know any associations with choanal atresia?

Answers to Question 6

6.1 What is your differential diagnosis?

- Unilateral choanal atresia
- CSF leak
- Antrochoanal polyp.

A full nasal examination, including anterior rhinoscopy and flexible nasendoscopy, should be performed. A CT scan of the sinuses would be a useful investigation.

6.2 CT scanning shows the following (see Figure 1.6.1). Tell me about this image.

This is an axial CT of the sinuses and shows right choanal atresia, with bony and membraneous (mixed) atresia. Patients can present late with a unilateral atresia, and would benefit from surgery to open this atretic segment. As this is a case of mixed atresia, a transnasal approach could be used.

6.3 How would you manage this patient?

This patient would benefit from surgically opening the atretic segment via a transnasal approach. The patient should be consented for complications, which include basi-sphenoid fracture, CSF leak, re-stenosis, and the need for serial dilatation.

Surgical technique for membranous atresia

- General anaesthesia, patient supine, reverse Trendelenburg position (head up)
- Prepare the nose with Moffats/lignocaine and adrenaline
- Using a Boyle–Davis gag and a 120-degree Hopkins rod endoscope, inspect the post-nasal space and atretic choana, whilst introducing a female urethral dilator to the affected nostril
- Direct the initial puncture (observed by seeing the mucosa blanch) towards the floor of the nose and the septum
- Without using excessive force, aim to dilate the airway as much as possible, taking care to avoid basi-sphenoid fracture.

For those with **bony atresia**, a diamond-burr drill can be used transnasally, using a speculum to guard the ala of the nostril. The palate must be observed to avoid puncture, and it is helpful to remove the posterior end of the septum (up to 7mm). The greater palatine and sphenopalatine arteries run laterally, and so aim to stay medial to avoid these. In an adult with unilateral atresia, stenting is not routinely required.

6.4 Do you know any associations with choanal atresia?

CHARGE

Neonates with bilateral choanal atresia will present with breathing difficulties, as they are obligate nasal breathers. The classic pattern is for respiratory distress, which improves on crying (the baby is breathing through the mouth). Eventually, a few hours after birth the baby tires and can develop respiratory failure. The inability to pass a nasogastric (NG) tube confirms the diagnosis, and an oral Guedel airway can be taped in position to maintain an airway. Surgical correction can then be arranged.

CHARGE is a non-random association of abnormalities including:

- Coloboma
- Heart abnormalities
- Atresia of the choana

- Retardation of growth and development
- Genitorenal abnormailites
- Ear malformations (such as Mondini anomaly, widened vestibular aqueduct and abnormal semicircular canals).

At least three major and three minor features should be present to confirm the diagnosis. It is an autosomal dominant defect of the *CHD7* gene.

Question 7

7.1 Describe the scans shown in Figures 1.7.1 and 1.7.2.

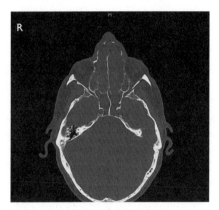

Figure 1.7.1

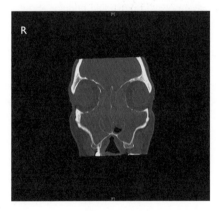

Figure 1.7.2

7.2 What is the management of bilateral nasal polyposis?

7.3 This patient has asthma. Is there anything else you would like to ask the patient in view of this? How might this change your management?

Answers to Question 7

7.1 Describe the scans shown in Figures 1.7.1 and 1.7.2.

These images show CT scans of the paranasal sinuses, one axial, the other coronal. They show soft tissue opacification of all of the sinuses and nasal cavity. This would be consistent with sinonasal polyposis. There is widening of the nasal bones suggesting long-standing disease.

7.2 What is the management of bilateral nasal polyposis?

Nasal polyps can be managed **medically** or **surgically**. For a patient with gross nasal polyps, oral prednisolone (for example, 40mg once daily for a week) may help to reduce the size to a tolerable level, which might then be maintained on topical nasal steroid.

However, those failing to respond, or requiring frequent oral steroids will benefit from **surgery** as an adjunct to medical therapies. The extent of the nasal surgery will depend on a number of factors, but will, at the very least, comprise a nasal polypectomy. In this situation, most surgeons would also undertake endoscopic sinus surgery (FESS), aiming to exenterate the ethmoid and maxillary sinuses.

The patient should understand that there is no definitive cure, and even with surgery they will need ongoing medical management to keep the polyps under control.

7.3 This patient has asthma. Is there anything else you would like to ask the patient in view of this? How might this change your management?

In any patient with bilateral nasal polyps, one should enquire about asthma and aspirin sensitivity (**Samter's triad**). These patients are difficult to control, have extensive polyposis, and recur quickly following surgery. They may benefit from a low salicylate diet, but it is difficult to exclude completely, as many foods contain a degree of salicylate. Wine, apples, potatoes, and olive oil are just a few foods containing high levels.

Other factors that may contribute to the development of nasal polyps include allergy (e.g. house dust mite), and infections. In children, **cystic fibrosis** and **Kartagener's syndrome** should be considered. Consider also Churg–Strauss syndrome.

Question 8

A 36-year-old female presents with diplopia, proptosis, and swelling over the left eye. This has been gradually been getting worse and now she has some discomfort over the area.

8.1 Figures 1.8.1 and 1.8.2 show CT scans. Describe them.

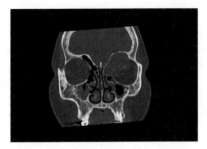

Figure 1.8.1

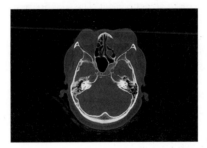

Figure 1.8.2

8.2 How do these develop?

8.3 How can they be treated?

8.4 How might you score/classify the sinus disease seen in this scan? How does this help you surgically?
Do you know of other grading systems used in assessing sinonasal CT scans? Why are these systems important?

8.5 What is likely to happen to the proptosis and diplopia in the long term?

Answers to Question 8

8.1 Figures 1.8.1 and 1.8.2 show CT scans. Describe them.

This is a CT of the sinuses showing axial and coronal cuts. The most obvious abnormality is a fronto-ethmoidal mucocoele, which is smooth, opacified, and is seen to displace the globe, accounting for the diplopia. There is thickening within the ethmoid and maxillary sinuses, and evidence of probably previous surgery, with large middle meatal antrostomies.

8.2 How do these develop?

When the dependent ostium of the frontal sinus is blocked, sterile mucus accumulates in the sinus. The cyst expands over time, causing the symptoms the patient has described, diplopia, and proptosis. If the cyst is infected it is termed a **pyocoele** and can be painful. Over time, the expanded cyst wall becomes very thin, and can be opened surgically to drain the cyst.

8.3 How can they be treated?

Surgical drainage

This can be done endoscopically, preparing the patient as for endoscopic sinus surgery. This patient's CT scan shows the middle turbinate attached directly to the dependent part of the mucocoele and lateral cribriform plate; this will make access difficult. The superior and medial border of the maxillary sinus will need to be removed to allow access to the mucocoele.

8.4 How might you score/classify the sinus disease seen in this scan? How does this help you surgically? Do you know of other grading systems used in assessing sinonasal CT scans? Why are these systems important?

There are several scoring systems for grading sinus disease; see Boxes 1.8.1 and 1.8.2.

Box 1.8.1 Lund and Mackay grading system

Each of the sinuses (maxillary, anterior/posterior ethmoids, frontal, and sphenoidal) are graded 0–2, where:

0 = clear

1 = partial opacification

2 = complete opacification.

The osteomeatal complex is graded separately where 0 = clear and 2 = obstructed (there is no '1' score). The maximum score is therefore 24. This is largely a tool for research, but in clinical practice, the higher the score the more confident one can be of sinus disease.

Staging reproduced from Lund V, MacKay V. 'Staging in rhinosinusitis'. *Rhinology* **107**,183–4. Copyight 1993, with permission of The International Rhinologic Society.

Box 1.8.2 **Keros Classification of the ethmoid roof**

- Type 1 olfactory fossa 1–3mm deep
- Type 2 olfactory fossa 4–7mm deep
- Type 3 olfactory fossa 8–16mm
- Type 4 (not in the original classification, but discussed in Stamberger's work on paranasal nomenclature) is used to describe olfactory fossa with asymmetric skull base.

From Type 1 to Type 4, there is an increasing chance of inadvertent intracranial injury.

Classification reproduced from Keros P (1962). Über die praktische Bedeutung der Niveauunterschiede der lamina cribrosa des ethmoids. *Z Laryngol Rhinol Otol* **41**: 808–13.

A useful mnemonic can be used as an *aide* memoire for describing CT scans before surgery; this ensures that important features are not missed:

'CLOSET'

C—cribriform plate

L—lamina

O—optic nerve/Onodi cells

S—sphenoid

E—ethmoid artery (Kennedy's nipple)

T—teeth.

8.5 What is likely to happen to the proptosis and diplopia in the long term?

The diplopia and proptosis are likely to improve over time, with bony remodelling after the surgical drainage.

Question 9

A teenage boy presents to the clinic with a history of progressive left-sided nasal obstruction and recurrent epistaxis. His parents feel that his left cheek is becoming swollen. His GP has performed a clotting screen, which was normal. He has tried a course of Naseptin, which has not helped.

9.1 What is your differential diagnosis?

9.2 On examination you find a large unilateral nasal mass. How would you confirm the diagnosis?

9.3 Your imaging confirms your suspicions. What are the options now?

Answers to Question 9

9.1 What is your differential diagnosis?

The most likely diagnosis is a **juvenile nasal angiofibroma** (JNA). This is a benign but aggressive tumour, which is has fibrous and vascular components arising from the region of the sphenoplatine foramen. They occur exclusively in adolescent male and their development may be related to hormonal changes around puberty.

This case is likely to be advanced as there is cheek swelling, which can be a sign that the pterygoid fossa is involved as the tumour extends around the maxilla. Although benign, there can be life-threatening haemorrhage, and extension into important local structures, such as ethmoid region (with eye effects), and intracranial extension. The location makes surgical excision challenging.

9.2 On examination you find a large unilateral nasal mass. How would you confirm the diagnosis?

Biopsy is contra-indicated because of the risk of bleeding. Urgent cross-sectional scanning in the form of CT and MRI scanning should be performed to ascertain the extent of the lesion and confirm the diagnosis. Classic findings on CT include

- Widening of the sphenopalatine foramen
- Bowing of the posterior maxillary sinus wall anteriorly (Holman–Miller sign)
- Bowing of the pterygoid plates posteriorly.

9.3 Your imaging confirms your suspicions. What are the options now?

The **Radkowski classification** (see Box 1.9.1) is used to grade JNA tumours.

Box 1.9.1 Radkowski classification

IA   Limited to nose and/or nasopharyngeal vault.
IB   Extension into ≥1 sinus.
IIA Minimal extension into PMF.
IIB Full occupation of PMF with or without erosion of orbital bones.
IIC Or posterior to pterygoid plates
IIIA Erosion of skull base—minimal intracranial extension.
IIIB Erosion of skull base—extensive intracranial extension with or without cavernous sinus invasion.

Classification reproduced from Radkowski D, McGill T, Healy GB, Ohlms L, Jones DT. Angiofibroma. Changes in staging and treatment. *Arch Otolaryngol Head Neck Surg* 1996;**122**:122–129.

The treatment of choice is surgical excision. Whatever approach is adopted, it is now standard practice to undertake preoperative embolization to reduce the risk of severe bleeding peri-operatively.

Approaches include:

- Endoscopic for small tumours
- Lateral rhinotomy
- Mid-facial degloving
- Transpalatal
- Caudwell–Luc
- Maxillary swing
- Craniofacial resection.

Radiotherapy may be used for inoperable/recurrent disease.

Question 10

A middle aged male presents with enopthalmos and left cheek pain, with a subjective sensation of left-sided nasal congestion.

10.1 Describe the imaging shown in Figures 1.10.1–1.10.3.

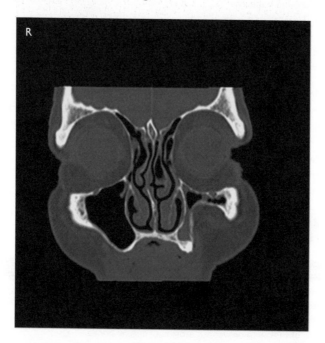

Figure 1.10.1

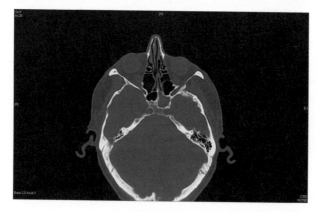

Figure 1.10.2

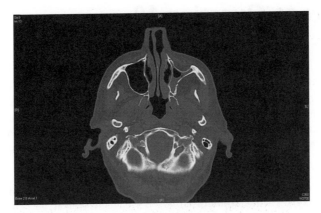

Figure 1.10.3

10.2 What is the diagnosis?

10.3 How would you manage this patient?

Answers to Question 10

10.1 Describe the imaging shown in Figures 1.10.1–1.10.3.

This is a series of CT images of the sinuses in the axial and coronal planes. They show enopthalmos, a small shrunken left maxillary sinus with the floor of the sinus elevated compared with the other side. The maxillary sinus is also partially opacified with air bubbles present. The osteomeatal complex is obstructed. The left middle turbinate has a concha bullosa and is paradoxical in its orientation.

10.2 What is the diagnosis?

These features are consistent with **silent sinus syndrome** (also known as **imploding maxillary sinus** or **maxillary sinus atelectasis**). In this acquired condition, the osteomeatal complex is obstructed and the maxillary sinus gradually reduces in size and is remodelled, 'imploding' on itself. Typically, all four walls of the sinus are retracted. The orbital wall is always retracted and commonly thinned.

10.3 How would you manage this patient?

The treatment is to restore normal sinus drainage by enlarging the maxillary ostium with endoscopic sinus surgery. Alternatively, an inferior meatal antrostomy can be used to re-aerate the sinus if access to the osteomeatal complex is challenging. In this patient, to access the ostromeatal complex, the concha bullosa would need to be excised. Limited resection of the middle turbinate might be required for access.

In patients with diplopia or severe cosmetic deformity, repair of the orbital floor may be required.

Question 11

A 30-year-old Afro-Caribbean lady presents to the clinic with whistling on breathing through her nose. She also admits to some crustiness and blocked sensation within the nose and has recently suffered malaise and some shortness of breath on exertion.

You examine this lady's nose and see a crusty perforation of the anterior septum (see Figure 1.11.1).

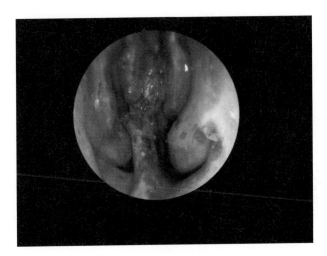

Figure 1.11.1

11.1 How would you manage this patient?

11.2 What tests would you do and why?

11.3 In general terms, what are the options for dealing with a septal perforation?

Answers to Question 11

11.1 How would you manage this patient?

The history should focus on:

- Nasal trauma
- Previous surgery
- Recreational drug use
- Systemic symptoms, such as weight loss, cough, urinary symptoms, sweats, and skin rashes/nodules.

The causes of a septal perforation can be:

- Traumatic (physical (e.g. nose-picking, surgery) or chemical)
- Infective (such as TB, syphilis)
- Inflammatory
- Neoplastic.

The history in this case suggests an inflammatory cause with systemic features.

Inflammatory conditions associated with septal perforations include Wegener's disease, sarcoidosis, systemic lupus erythematosus (SLE) and polyarteritis nodosa (PAN).

Sarcoidosis is the most likely diagnosis here. It is a non-caseating granulomatous disease, commonly affecting young adults. Afro-Caribbeans are more often affected and more severely, frequently with extra-thoracic disease. Sarcoidosis may also be characterized by *lupus pernio*, with raised indurated skin lesions affecting the skin of the nose, cheeks, lips, hands, fingers, and forehead.

11.2 What tests would you do and why?

This patient requires a battery of blood tests, chest X-ray (CXR), CT sinuses.

The blood tests would include those shown in Table 1.11.1.

FBC	To rule out	Anaemia
ESR	To rule out	Inflammation
U&E	To rule out	Renal compromise
cANCA	To rule out	Wegener's, (non-caseating granulomatous vasculitis of small to medium vessels). cANCA is highly specific in the acute phase (90%), but only positive in 60% of those with isolated nasal disease
ACE levels	To rule out	Sarcoid (ACE level corresponds to disease activity)
Calcium		This can be raised in sarcoid
CXR	To rule out	Upper lobe fibrosis/bilateral hilar lymphadenopathy in sarcoid
CT sinuses	To rule out	Sinusitis, extent and shows any bone destruction

cANCA, cytoplasmic antineutrophil cytoplasmic antibody; ESR, erythrocyte sedimentation rate; U&E, urea & electrolytes; ACE, angiotensin-converting enzyme.

Table 1.11.1 Blood tests recommended

A **biopsy** of the perforation should be performed.

11.3 In general terms, what are the options for dealing with a septal perforation?

Conservative management

If there is an underlying medical cause, treat this in liaison with rheumatology colleagues.

If the patient is left with residual symptoms, such as bleeding or crusting, simply suggest the use of saline douches and petroleum jelly. Intermittent nasal creams, such as naseptin may also be required.

Surgical options

These include placing a silastic button in the defect. This will reduce whistling, crusting, and bleeding, and is well tolerated by most patients. Surgical repairs can be attempted using septal mucosal flaps, or even cartilage grafts harvested from the pinna, but results are variable, especially in a patient with underlying inflammatory disease, and complication and failure rates are high.

Question 12

12.1 What flap is being planned for this patient (see Figure 1.12.1)?

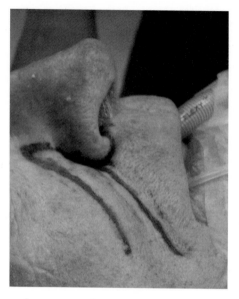

Figure 1.12.1

12.2 How would you describe this flap and what is the blood supply to it?

12.3 Give some examples of uses for this flap?

12.4 Discuss the advantages and disadvantages of using this flap to repair a full thickness defect of the alar rim.

Answers to Question 12

12.1 What flap is being planned for this patient (see Figure 1.12.1)?

The image shows the planning stages for a nasolabial flap.

12.2 How would you describe this flap and what is the blood supply to it?

This is an axial pattern flap, which receives its blood supply from branches of the facial artery, the angular artery. A superiorly based flap can also be raised.

12.3 Give some examples of uses for this flap?

- This flap can be used to repair the lateral nasal wall
- It can also be used intra-orally to repair floor of mouth defects
- Collumella repairs
- Upper lip repairs.

12.4 Discuss the advantages and disadvantages of using this flap to repair a full thickness defect of the alar rim.

Advantages

- Good skin colour and texture matching to the nose. The cheek area is usually non-hair bearing
- Robust flap, and a large area of skin can be raised
- Can be done under local anaesthetic (LA)
- Primary closure of the donor site is usually possible
- Minimal donor site cosmetic deformity.

Disadvantages

- A full thickness defect implies loss of cartilage, which this flap will not replace so collapse of the alar margin may occur
- The skin can be very thick giving a poor cosmetic appearance.

Question 13

A 50-year-old male patient presents to the ear, nose, and throat (ENT) clinic with unilateral nasal obstruction.

13.1 What questions are pertinent in the history?

13.2 Describe your examination technique.

13.3 It is evident that he has a unilateral nasal mass (see Figure 1.13.1). What investigations would be appropriate?

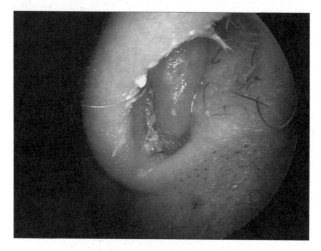

Figure 1.13.1 Unilateral nasal mass.

13.4 Describe the CT scans shown in Figures 1.13.2 and 1.13.3. What is the differential diagnosis here?

13.5 What is the next appropriate course of action?

13.6 What are the clinical and pathological features of inverted papilloma?

13.7 What is the management of inverted papilloma?

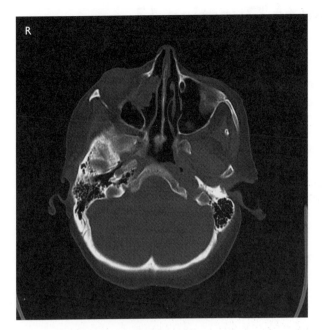

Figure 1.13.2

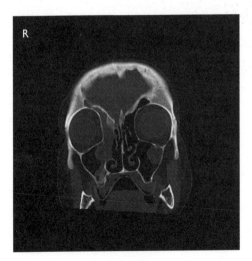

Figure 1.13.3

Answers to Question 13

13.1 What questions are pertinent in the history?

The history should focus on:

- Duration of symptoms
- Epistaxis
- Fluctuation in obstruction
- Pain
- Eye symptoms (diplopia, epiphora, pain on movement, change in acuity)
- Smoking and tobacco usage
- Occupational history (hardwood workers are at increased risk of ethmoid adenocarcinoma; workers in the nickel and leather industries are also at risk of sinonasal cancer).

13.2 Describe your examination technique.

Apply nasal decongestant and/or local anaesthetic. Start with anterior rhinoscopy with a Thudichum speculum. Proceed to nasal endoscopy (rigid or fibre-optic), concentrating on a 'three-pass' technique—above middle turbinate, in the middle meatus, and in the inferior meatus. Be sure to inspect the post-nasal space.

Examine the oral cavity (antro-choanal polyp can prolapse into the oropharynx). Finally, bearing in mind that malignancy is a possibility in this case, examine the neck.

13.3 It is evident that he has a unilateral nasal mass (see Figure 1.13.1). What investigations would be appropriate?

In the first instance, a CT scan of the paranasal sinuses would suffice.

13.4 Describe the CT scans shown in Figures 1.13.2 and 1.13.3. What is the differential diagnosis here?

These are CT scans of the paranasal sinuses in the coronal and axial planes. They show soft tissue density opacification of the middle meatus extending towards the frontal recess. Of note, there are some small areas of calcification of the soft tissue mass. This suggests either fungal disease or inverted papilloma. Malignancy is also a possibility in this case.

13.5 What is the next appropriate course of action?

A tissue biopsy is required for histological examination.

13.6 What are the clinical and pathological features of inverted papilloma?

Inverted papilloma (Schneiderian papilloma or Ringertz tumour) is a benign tumour of the nasal cavity. The tumours typically arise on the lateral nasal wall in the middle meatus. Although the tumours are benign, they are locally expansile and occasionally destructive.

Radiologically, the tumour is seen to arise from the area of the middle meatus, and can often expand the maxillary ostium. The tumour itself may demonstrate calcification. Adjacent bone may be thinned, eroded or sclerotic. Thus, the radiological features are not dissimilar to malignancy. MRI scanning may be helpful: it can help to differentiate tumour from inflammatory tissue. In addition, the MRI will show a feature known as **convoluted cerebriform pattern**, in which alternating parallel lines of high and low intensity are seen within the tumour.

Histologically, they are characterized by ribbons of respiratory epithelium enclosed by basement membrane, which grows into the subjacent stroma (thus with an inverted pattern) with characteristic micro-mucous cysts. Up to 10% may demonstrate dysplasia, and there is a small group that undergo malignant degeneration.

Adequate surgical exision is curative. Long-term follow-up needs to be maintained to monitor for recurrence and to deal with any nasal crusting that arises.

13.7 What is the management of inverted papilloma?

Complete surgical exision is curative, so this is the aim of treatment. Small- to moderate-sized tumours may be approached endoscopically. Recent advances in endoscopic equipment mean that a fairly extensive endoscopic medial maxillectomy may be performed endoscopically.

Very large tumours, however, will require an open approach. Either a mid-facial degloving or a lateral rhinotomy may be performed, according to the surgeon's preference and expertise.

Whichever approach is employed, the resultant cavity must be easy to inspect endoscopically to allow for post-operative surveillance.

Question 14

A 42-year-old gentleman presents to the ophthalmologists with a 1-week history of a swollen left eyelid and ipsilateral nasal discharge. The ophthalmologists have attempted to aspirate what they presume to be a simple skin abscess of his left eyelid They are able to drain some pus, but ask the ENT surgeons for an opinion.

14.1 What questions are relevant in the history?

14.2 How should the clinical examination proceed?

In the course of your conversation with him, it is evident that the patient is drowsy and confused. He was previously fit and well.

14.3 What is the next appropriate course of action?

14.4 The CT scans are shown in Figures 1.14.1–1.14.3. Describe the findings.

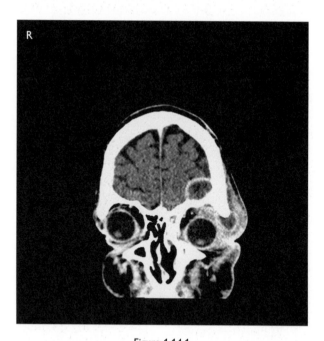

Figure 1.14.1

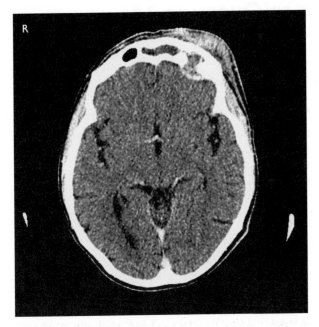

Figure 1.14.2

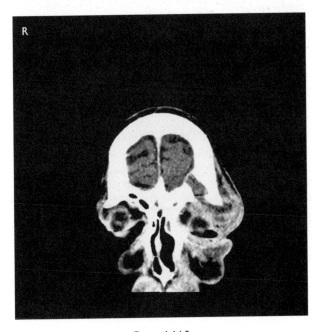

Figure 1.14.3

14.5 Based on the situation now, how would you proceed?

Answers to Question 14

14.1 What questions are relevant in the history?

The history should cover:

- Duration of current symptoms
- Nature of current rhinorrhoea—mucky, clear?
- Past history of sinusitis
- Previous history of nasal discharge/obstruction/rhinorrhoea
- Previous sinus surgery
- Skin trauma (bites/scratches/abrasions)
- Any suggestion of immunocompromise.

14.2 How should the clinical examination proceed?

Apply nasal decongestant and/or local anaesthetic. Start with anterior rhinoscopy with a Thudichum speculum. Proceed to nasal endoscopy (rigid or fibre-optic), concentrating on a 'three-pass' technique—above middle turbinate, in the middle meatus, and in the inferior meatus. Be sure to inspect the post-nasal space. Make particular note of any pus or polyps arising from the middle meatus.

If possible, perform an eye examination—test pupillary reflexes, eye movements (asking about pain or diplopia), acuity, and colour vision.

14.3 What is the next appropriate course of action?

Given the deterioration in his conscious state, there is a concern that he has an intracranial complication. Further medical support should be requested, adequate venous access achieved, and intravenous antibiotics commenced.

An urgent CT of his sinuses and head (with contrast) should be arranged. Given that he is likely to need surgical intervention, he should be kept nil-by-mouth.

The neurosurgeons should be consulted.

14.4 The CT scans are shown in Figures 1.14.1–3. Describe the findings.

This CT scan shows the presence of an intracranial abscess as a result of frontal sinusitis. On the axial scan, a breach of the posterior wall of the left frontal sinus is clearly seen communicating with the extradural abscess. The floor of the frontal sinus is also eroded, and the abscess has tracked anteriorly and laterally into the upper eyelid, hence, the clinical appearance.

14.5 Based on the situation now, how would you proceed?

This is a complex case requiring expert neurosurgical input. If the patient is not yet in a neurosurgical centre, his immediate transfer should be arranged.

The priority is on drainage of the abscess. The exact approach to this should be discussed with the neurosurgical team, but it is likely that all three components of the abscess (sinus, intracranial, eyelid) could be drained through a single incision in the forehead.

Chapter 2

Head and neck

Question 1

This patient presents 15 months after his original laryngectomy surgery with pain, bleeding, and swelling around his stoma (see Figures 2.1.1 and 2.1.2).

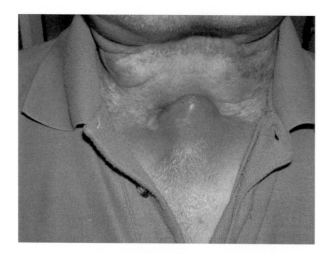

Figure 2.1.1

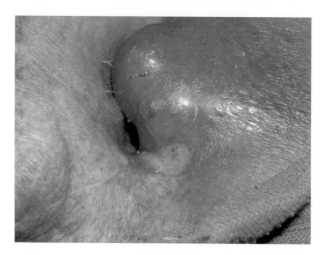

Figure 2.1.2

1.1 What is the likely diagnosis and how would you confirm it?

1.2 What are the pre-operative factors that predispose to this complication?

1.3 What is the relevant classification system?

1.4 What are the management options in this condition?

1.5 How should *this* patient be managed?

Answers to Question 1

1.1 What is the likely diagnosis and how would you confirm it?

The mass shown is highly suspicious of a stomal recurrence of squamous cell carcinoma. Diagnosis will usually be confirmed with fine needle aspiration (FNA) cytology. A CT/magnetic resonance imaging (MRI) will usually be required to stage extent.

1.2 What are the pre-operative factors that predispose to this complication?

Tumour factors

The risk of stomal recurrence increases largely as a result of the adequacy of excision and the risk of para-tracheal lymph node involvement.
- More advanced tumours
- Positive tracheal resection margin
- Transglottic and subglottic tumours
- Laryngeal cartilage invasion
- Tumour spread via the crico-thyroid membrane
- Pre and para-tracheal (level 7) node involvement
- Level 4 lymph node metastases
- Salvage laryngectomy after radiotherapy.

Pre-operative tracheostomy

Patients presenting with stridor and requiring a tracheostomy pre-operatively have been shown to be associated with as increased risk of stomal recurrence (8–26%). Two theories may explain this finding:

1. Implantation of tumour cells during tracheostomy into the skin and para-tracheal tissues
2. Patients requiring a tracheostomy, by definition have advanced disease and, hence, are more at risk of having involved para-tracheal nodal metastases.

The risk of stomal recurrence is reduced by performing subsequent laryngectomy within 48h of initial tracheostomy. However, Narula et al. (1993) found that emergency laryngectomy (within 24h of tracheostomy) conferred no overall survival advantage ultimately.

1.3 What is the relevant classification system?

Sisson described:
- Type 1—localized. Usually discreet nodule in *superior* aspect of stoma
- Type 2—*Oesophageal* involvement. No inferior extension
- Type 3—*Inferior* to stoma. Usually mediastinal extension
- Type 4—*Lateral* extension. +/− Carotid sheath involvement.

1.4 What are the management options in this condition?

Curative

- *Radical surgery*—only consider this if sufficient surgical margins can be predicted. Aim to excise the lesion in continuity with an ellipse of skin around stoma. Thoracic surgery may be required in order to access the upper mediastinum and great vessels. Excision of the manubrium, medial ends of both clavicles with mobilization of the trachea and formation of a new low tracheostomy. Excise lymph nodes, thyroid remnant, neopharynx, and skin as necessary. Use regional skin flaps, or pedicled pectoralis major, or latissimus dorsi flaps. If neopharyngo-oesophagectomy is required, consider stomach transposition or free jejunal transfer for total pharyngeal reconstruction.
- *Radiotherapy*, if this has not been given previously. However, in most patients requiring laryngectomy (and with positive risk factors for stomal recurrence) this will already have been given.

Palliative

Manage airway restriction:

- Tracheostomy tube
- Steroids
- *Debulking of tumour*—CO_2 laser or microdebrider
- *Brachytherapy*—iridium-192 wire spiralling around outer part of a tracheotomy tube.

General palliative care issues

Symptom control, e.g. pain, involve palliative care team.

1.5 How should *this* patient be managed?

- Multi-disciplinary team (MDT) discussion
- Evaluate extent of local disease with CT/MRI neck +/− rigid endoscopy
- Exclude distant metastatic disease. CT neck and chest
- Medical work up—is patient fit for surgery?
- Discuss the options with patient and family.

Further reading

Narula AA, Shepard IJ, West K, Bradley PJ (1993). Is emergency laryngectomy a waste of time? *Am J Otolaryngol* **14:** 21–3.

Question 2

2.1 Describe the phases of swallowing.

2.2 Give an account of the neurology of swallowing.

2.3 Describe the management options in a 60-year-old patient with unilateral vocal cord palsy of neurological origin and aspiration.

Answers to Question 2

2.1 Describe the phases of swallowing.

Definition

Swallowing (deglutition)—the process that normally involves the passage of food from the mouth to the stomach via the oesophagus.

3 phases—oral, pharyngeal, oesophageal (see Figure 2.2.1).

Oral phase (voluntary)

- *Oral preparatory phase* (Fig 2.2.1a)
  - ◆ Mastication and addition and mixing of saliva to form a food bolus held anterolaterally against the hard palate by the tongue
  - ◆ Requires the taste, temperature, touch, and proprioception senses for formation of a bolus of the right size and consistency
- *Oral transit phase (1s)* (Fig 2.2.1b and c)
  - ◆ Elevation of the anterior tongue as it meets the hard palate to push the food bolus posteriorly into the pharynx to commence the pharyngeal phase
  - ◆ Requires that a labial seal be maintained to prevent food from leaking from the mouth, and a buccal musculature tension to prevent food from getting into the recess between the mandible and cheek.

Pharyngeal phase (involuntary, 1s)

- See Fig 2.2.1d and e
- Triggered at anterior tonsillar pillar
- Retraction of the tongue and nasophayngeal closure with palate elevation (levator and tensor veli palatini) and contraction of superior constrictor
- Deglutition apnoea
- Glottic closure with approximation of true vocal cords, false vocal cords, and aryepiglottic folds to the epiglottis (in order)
- Laryngeal elevation through action of supra-hyoid strap muscles and thyro-hyoid, resulting in epiglottic rotation to 60° below horizontal and relaxation of cricopharyngeus, allowing the bolus to pass into the oesophagus.

Oesophageal phase (involuntary, 8–20s)

- See Fig 2.2.1f
- Under the control of the brain stem and the myenteric plexus. A peristaltic wave beginning in the pharynx pushes the bolus sequentially from the cervical oesophagus down through the relaxed lower oesophageal sphincter into the stomach
- Resumption of expiration.

2.2 Give an account of the neurology of swallowing.

The process of swallowing is organized with sensory input from receptors in the base of the tongue, soft palate, tonsillar arches, tonsils, and the posterior pharyngeal wall, via the lingual (VII), glossopharyngeal (IX), and laryngeal nerves (X) to the swallowing centre located within the pontine reticular system.

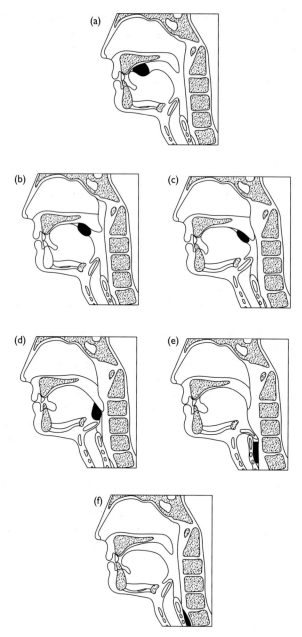

Figure 2.2.1 The phases of swallowing. Reproduced from the *Oxford Handbook of Clinical Rehabilitation*, 2nd edn. Anthony Ward, Michael Barnes, Sandra Stark, Sarah Ryan, copyright 2009 with permission of Oxford University Press.

Information from the swallowing centre then is conveyed back to the muscles that help in swallowing through trigeminal (V), facial (VII), glossopharyngeal (IX), laryngeal (X), and hypoglossal (XII) nerves via the trigeminal, facial, and hypoglossal motor nuclei and nucleus ambiguous.

- *CN V—trigeminal:*
  - Contains both sensory and motor fibres that innervate the face
  - Important for masticators, buccinators
- *CN VII—facial:*
  - Contains both sensory and motor fibres
  - Important for taste to anterior 2/3 of tongue (via lingual)
- *CN IX—glossopharyngeal:*
  - Contains both sensory and motor fibres
  - Important for sensation of oropharynx and taste to posterior 1/3 of tongue and sensation of the pharynx
- *CN X—vagus:*
  - Contains both sensory and motor fibres
  - Important for taste to oropharynx, and sensation and motor function to larynx and laryngopharynx (via superior and recurrent laryngeal nerves)
  - Important for airway protection
- *CN XII—hypoglossal:* contains motor fibres that primarily innervate the tongue.

2.3 Describe the management options in a 60-year-old patient with a unilateral vocal cord palsy of neurological origin and aspiration.

In the patient with dysphonia without significant aspiration, voice therapy can be used as sole treatment or as part of combined treatment. Patients with significant risk of aspiration pneumonia and treatment should commence promptly. Speech therapy assessment of the safety of the swallow is essential and where necessary Functional Endoscopic Evaluation of the Swallowing (FEES) or video-fluoroscopy may give useful information and help to quantify the risk. In addition, differing food consistencies and positions may be tried in order to find the optimal position and swallowing strategy.

- *Non-surgical:*
  - Oral feeding with consistency modifications
  - Compensatory strategies to reduce the risk of aspiration include chin tuck, head rotation (towards side of palsy), supraglottic swallow
  - NG/percutaneous endoscopic gastrostomy (PEG) feeding
- Surgical intervention may help to improve glottis closure and the efficacy of the cough, or prevent soiling of the lower respiratory tree. Rarely, it may be necessary to separate the airway from the digestive tract
  - Injection medialization laryngoplasty
  - Type I (Isshiki) thyroplasty
  - Tracheostomy
  - Laryngeal closure + tracheostomy
  - Tracheo-oesophageal diversion/laryngo-tracheal separation
  - Laryngectomy.

Question 3

This patient presents with a diffusely enlarged thyroid gland, deranged thyroid function tests and eyes as shown in Figure 2.3.1.

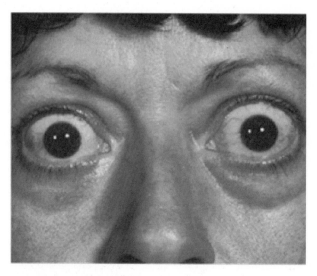

Figure 2.3.1 Reproduced from the *Oxford Handbook of Clinical Medicine,* 8th edn. Murray Longmore, Ian Wilkinson, Edward Davidson et al., copyright 2010 with permission of Oxford University Press.

3.1 What is the most likely diagnosis and how would you confirm this?

3.2 What are the options for treating Graves' disease?

3.3 What are the indications for surgery in this case?

3.4 What is the major life threatening surgical complication with hyperthyroid patients?

3.5 What are its clinical features?

3.6 How is it managed?

3.7 How do you prepare a thyrotoxic patient for surgery?

3.8 What is the surgery of choice?

3.9 What are the potential complications?

3.10 What are the early symptoms of hypocalcaemia?

3.11 How do you manage it?

3.12 What is the role of vitamin D replacement?

3.13 What other effects does the loss of the parathyroids have?

Answers to Question 3

3.1 What is the most likely diagnosis and how would you confirm this?

The clinical picture fits with a diagnosis of Graves' disease. This can be confirmed with a thyroid auto-antibody screen.

3.2 What are the options for treating Graves' disease?

- Medical
  - ◆ Beta blockade, reverses the thyrotoxic symptoms in 12–24h, it also may inhibit T4 to T3 conversion
  - ◆ *Carbimazole*—is metabolized to the biologically active methimazole and blocks iodination of tyrosine required in thyroxine production. This takes 3–4 weeks to take effect. When given for 12–18 months, more than 50% relapse. Other side effects include agranulocytosis, arthralgia, and rash
  - ◆ *Propylthiouracil*—also blocks tyrosine iodination and T4 to T3 conversion and works faster than carbimazole
- Radioiodine ablation I^{131}, concentrates in metabolically active thyroid tissue so destroying any functioning cells in 6–10 weeks. Hypothyroidism can occur years later and is contraindicated in pregnancy
- Surgery will commonly comprise a total thyroidectomy.

3.3 What are the indications for surgery in this case?

In patients who are fit for surgery and where:
- The symptoms are not responsive to long-term antithyroid drug therapy or where toxic side effects have occurred
- Patients who are deemed unsuitable for radioiodine ablation, e.g. pregnancy
- Severe exophthalmos
- Huge gland with airway obstruction
- Suspicion of carcinoma on fine needle aspiration cytology (FNAC).

3.4 What is the major life threatening surgical complication with hyperthyroid patients?

Thyroid storm: this is usually abrupt and precipitated by stress, e.g. surgery or infection.

3.5 What are its clinical features?

The features are a function of a marked increase in the metabolic rate due to rapid release of thyroid hormones, i.e. fever, increased CO_2 production, acidosis, hyperventilation, tachycardia, arrhythmia, cardiac failure, shock, agitation, delirium, coma, abdominal pain, vomiting, and diarrhoea.

3.6 How is it managed?

Thyroid storm is a life-threatening emergency and where suspected do not wait for laboratory confirmation before starting treatment. Therapy should include active cooling, beta blockade (propranolol 1–5mg IV), Glucocorticoid (possible adrenocortical exhaustion), IV Iodide (KI 60mg bd or NaI 1–2.5mg) or lithium. Do not give aspirin as this displaces T4 from thyroid-binding globulin, so making the situation worse. Admit the patient to ITU and urgently involve the endocrinology team.

3.7 How do you prepare a thyrotoxic patient for surgery?

This is best done in multidisciplinary setting with discussion an endocrinologist, surgeon and anaesthetist. Where possible pharmacological stabilization will require 6–8 weeks of beta blockade in combination with iodine or lithium administration. Using these treatment patients can usually be rendered euthyroid in 1–2 weeks, however, the cardiac effects can take longer to resolve.

3.8 What is the surgery of choice?

One stage total thyroidectomy reduces the recurrence rate and seems to reduce anti-thyroid autoimmunity as well as reducing any exacerbation of ophthalmoplegia.

3.9 What are the potential complications?

- Haematoma and wound infection
- 1–2% permanent hypoparathyoidism
- 1–4% recurrence of hyperthyroidism.
- 1% laryngeal nerve injury
- 10% transient post-operative hypocalcaemia.

3.10 What are the early symptoms of hypocalcaemia?

Circumoral tingling, paraesthesia, Chvostek's sign, Trousseau's sign (carpopedal spasm).

3.11 How do you manage it?

Confirm with serum Ca if possible. Start 10ml 10% calcium gluconate IV over 5–10min, until symptoms subside. If corrected calcium is less than 1.8mmol/l (even if asymptomatic) start Ca gluconate infusion. Once stable commence oral calcium. The aim is to maintain corrected calcium level between 2–2.3mmol/l.

3.12 What is the role of vitamin D replacement?

Some give vitamin D straight away while other practitioners argue that it makes the control of calcium levels more difficult and increases the chance of hypercalcaemia, as the hypocalcaemia is often transient.

1 α-hydroxycholecalciferol (alfacalcidol) 2μg is given daily or as Calcichew D3 (combined with calcium). It is activated in the liver to 1.25 dihydroxycholecalciferol, which increases uptake of calcium in the gut and reabsorption in the kidney.

3.13 What other effects does the loss of the parathyroids have?

There is decreased magnesium and increased phosphate serum concentrations.

Question 4

An otherwise fit 59-year-old man presented to the ENT clinic 1 week ago with an asymptomatic lump in the right neck. The mass measured approximately 7cm. A full ENT examination did not reveal any other pathology and an FNA and CT scan of his neck and chest were organized. He now returns to see you with the results of these investigations. The CT scan shows no chest disease and normal appearances of the upper aero-digestive tract. The cytology confirms squamous cell carcinoma.

4.1 What is the diagnosis and what do you think the probable tumour, nodes, metastasis (TNM) stage is?

4.2 What other investigations may be considered in this case and what is their rationale?

4.3 Assuming no primary is found discuss the treatment options for this patient (both surgical and non-surgical).

Answers to Question 4

4.1 What is the diagnosis and what do you think the probable TNM stage is?

This patient has metastatic squamous cell carcinoma affecting the right level 2/3 node with an unknown primary. Given that this is over 6cm in diameter, it is an N3 node. The overall stage therefore is T0 (previously Tx), N3, M0.

4.2 What other investigations may be considered in this case and what is their rationale?

The focus of further investigation is to try and identify an occult primary site, which in this case is likely to be tonsil or tongue base with pyriform fossa and nasopharynx being less likely. An **MRI** scan would provide superior soft tissue definition to the CT already performed, and any asymmetry noted in these sites would require biopsy.

Where available in a timely fashion a PET CT is likely to be the best investigation. Grade 3 evidence from observational studies has shown that it may identify 1 in 3 of occult primaries. In order to avoid any false positive results PET CT should be performed before any biopsies are taken.

Panendoscopy and biopsy will also be required in order make a tissue diagnosis from any suspicious sites shown on the investigations thus far. A complete examination of the upper aero-digestive tract should be performed including palpation of the oral cavity, tongue base, and tonsil. If no primary site is identified, ipsilateral blind biopsies of the post nasal space, tongue base, +/– pyriform fossa and at least an ipsilateral tonsillectomy should be performed. Increased reporting of positive biopsies from contra lateral tonsillectomy in this group of patients has led to bilateral tonsillectomy becoming routine practice in the unknown primary.

4.3 Assuming no primary is found discuss the treatment options for this patient (both surgical and non-surgical).

This patient's treatment options should be discussed as part of a head and neck MDT taking into account the patient's comorbidities and wishes. Treatment offered to this patient is likely to be with curative intent although the prognosis may be guarded given the extent of the nodal disease.

This is a relatively rare group of patients meaning there is limited evidence to direct best practice.

Such a patient with bulky neck disease will be treated effectively with combination surgery and (chemo) radiotherapy. Surgery will involve an ipsilateral modified radical neck dissection, with a contralateral selective neck dissection in addition if this was felt to be at risk on imaging.

The patient should undergo post-operative radiotherapy to the neck; however, the more difficult decision is whether to irradiate all the potential mucosal primary sites as this is associated with significantly increased morbidity. In some units where the nasopharynx is PET CT and biopsy negative this site may be spared from irradiation since the morbidity from irradiation is high.

The role of induction chemotherapy as a primary treatment is expanding and offers a viable alternative treatment strategy, particularly where the disease is thought to be human papilloma virus (HPV) related. Salvage surgery is then appropriate in those with an incomplete response.

Question 5

5.1 Describe your assessment and investigations in a 68-year-old male patient presenting with a 6-month history of voice change and who, on examination, is found to have a left vocal cord palsy (see Figure 2.5.1).

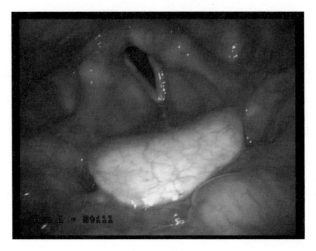

Figure 2.5.1

5.2 How would you manage a similar patient where the vocal abnormality occurred immediately following thyroid surgery, where the recurrent laryngeal nerve (RLN) was seen and preserved? (Assume that you are seeing the patient 3 weeks after their operation.).

5.3 The same patient remains symptomatic and the RLN shows no signs of recovery after 1 year. How would you advise and manage the patient?

Answers to Question 5

5.1 Describe your assessment and investigations in a 68 year old male patient presenting with a 6-month history of voice change and who, on examination, is found to have a left vocal cord palsy (see Figure 2.5.1).

The concern here is of malignant infiltration of the recurrent laryngeal nerve; hence primary investigations should be targeted to excluding this as a cause.

Take a full history—enquiring particularly about and respiratory, swallowing, or other neurological symptoms.

Perform a full ENT examination—including nasolaryngoscopy and note the size of the glottic gap during phonation and cranio-caudal position of the cord. Perform a full neck examination paying particular attention to the thyroid gland. If available a video-stroboscopic examination would be also be desirable.

Baseline blood screening tests include—FBC, U&Es, TFTs, CRP and viral serology and request an **immediate CXR**—looking for a large primary lung cancer. If the CXR is normal then move on to:

Secondary investigations

- CT from skull base to the diaphragm assessing the entire course of the RLN
- Panendoscopy gives the advantage that the arytenoid may be palpated to distinguish vocal cord palsy from cricoarytenoid fixation.

Occasionally, laryngeal electromyography may be required to differentiate between a unilateral vocal fold paralysis and cricoarytenoid joint pathology.

Other investigations may include a barium swallow and/or thyroid ultrasound scan depending upon the clinical picture.

5.2 How would you manage a similar patient where the vocal abnormality occurred immediately following thyroid surgery, where the RLN was seen and preserved? (Assume that you are seeing the patient 3 weeks after their operation).

Possible causes

RLN neuropraxia, RLN wrongly identified and damaged intra-operatively or cricoarytenoid joint dislocation resulting from endotracheal intubation trauma

Management should begin with confirmation of the pre-operative vocal cord status, and ensure that the lesion was not pre-existing. Exclude wound haematoma. If there is a suggestion of arytenoid dislocation this should be confirmed by palpation under a general anaesthetic or laryngeal EMG. Where there is a RLN injury at this stage there is good chance of recovery/compensation with good vocal function. Hence treatment should be conservative with speech and language therapy input.

An alternative would be to perform an injection of a temporary filler to medialize the vocal cord, whilst awaiting recovery. This injection could either be performed under general anaesthetic (GA) or LA.

5.3 The same patient remains symptomatic and the RLN shows no signs of recovery after 1 year. How would you advise and manage the patient?

Assuming the patient has complied with speech and language therapy (SALT) then counsel the patient that spontaneous recovery is very unlikely to happen beyond this stage. Idiopathic palsy can sometimes recover after 2 years. EMG can be used to help predict recovery. If the patient wishes to consider surgery discuss vocal cord medialization surgery. The choice of which technique will depend on the patient's/surgeon's preference and experience as well as the vocal demands of the patient.

Surgical options

- *Local anaesthetic medialization thyroplasty*—advantages include control over vocal cord (VC) position with intra-operative feedback, less changes in vocal cord volume, mass or stiffness. The procedure may be reversed if function returns
- *Arytenoid adduction*—performed alone or adjunct to thyroplasty, this is useful if there is a large posterior glottic chink
- *Vocal cord injection medialization*—this can be performed via a percutaneous technique under LA or endoscopically under GA. Disadvantages here include cord changes in mass, stiffness and volume, difficulty in estimating the amount of medialization required to achieve optimal voice, distribution of the injected material and local reaction, e.g. granulation, which was problematic with Teflon, although modern equivalents suffer this complication less frequently.

Question 6

6.1 Describe Figure 2.6.1.

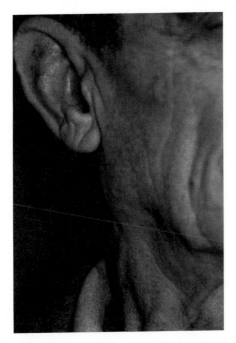

6.2 How (and why) would you investigate this patient?

6.3 What risks do you tell patients regarding parotid surgery?

6.4 Describe the methods of identifying the facial nerve in parotid surgery.

Answers to Question 6

6.1 Describe Figure 2.6.1.

This is a view of the right lateral side of the face showing a mass behind the angle of the mandible, below the mastoid tip and slightly displacing the lobule of the pinna. This is in keeping with a parotid mass, most likely a pleomorphic adenoma, though it could also be Warthin's tumour, adenocarcinoma, adenoidcystic carcinoma, lymph node or lymphoma. In this static view the facial nerve function appears normal.

6.2 How (and why) would you investigate this patient?

FNAC

Helps differentiate benign from malignant. It is a quick, cheap, and relatively easy procedure that can allay patients' anxiety and aids in their pre-operative counselling regarding the risk of facial nerve palsy, which would be low in benign lesions, but the risk is significantly increased in malignancy.

Radiology

CT or MRI scanning helps show extension to deep lobe, the choice of which depending on local availability and personnel preference. Imaging confirms that the mass is solitary, is confined to the parotid and will show the presence of a dumb-bell shaped tumour if it extends deeply to the parapharyngeal space.

6.3 What risks do you tell patients regarding parotid surgery?

- In experienced hands the risk of damage to the facial nerve and subsequent facial weakness is low (permanent <2%, temporary 15–20%)
- Gustatory sweating (Frey's syndrome) due to re-routing of parasympathetic secretomotor fibres (via auriculo-temporal nerve)
- Parasthesia of lower pinna/pre-auricular region (division of great auricular nerve)
- Haematoma
- Seroma
- Sailvary duct fistula
- Cosmetic change/scar.

6.4 Describe the methods of identifying the facial nerve in parotid surgery.

The main trunk of nerve can be found as it exits the skull base, before it enters the substance of the gland by its close relationship to the apex of the tragal cartilage, (cartilaginous pointer, when the ear is pulled posteriorly). The main trunk lies 1cm anterior, 1cm inferior, and 1cm deep. In addition the stylomastoid foramen (from which the facial nerve exits the skull) lies at the root of the tympano-mastoid fissure (sulcus). Furthermore, it may also be identified as it bisects the angle between the mastoid process and the posterior belly of the digastric (at the same depth as the superior surface of the muscle).

Once the main trunk of the nerve is identified the dissection can proceed forward to expose the nerve branching and defining the superficial and deep lobes of the parotid gland.

On occasions, defining the main trunk of the nerve may be difficult in which case individual branches maybe identified distally and traced proximally to the main trunk. Surface markings are as follows:

- *Marginal: mandibular*—1cm inferior to angle of mandible
- *Zygomatic*—crosses zygomatic arch at its mid-point, i.e. halfway along a line drawn between the lateral canthus and the tragus
- *Buccal*—1cm inferior and parallel to the parotid duct.

Very occasionally, it may be necessary to identify the facial nerve within the mastoid bone and follow its course as it exits the skull base.

Facial nerve monitoring and stimulation can also be used to help identify the nerve, but should not be relied upon as the only method.

Question 7

This 48-year-old patient presents with a 2-month history of a painful throat with some mild hoarseness of the voice. The symptoms seem to have been related to a preceding upper respiratory tract infection (URTI). The patient is a life-long non-smoker. Figure 2.7.1 shows the lesion as seen on laryngoscopy under GA.

7.1 What is the abnormality seen in Figure 2.7.1?

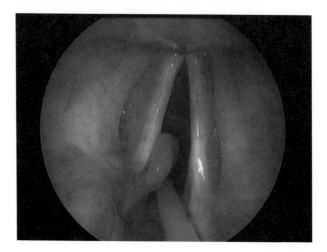

Figure 2.7.1

7.2 Give the differential diagnosis.

7.3 Give an account of the management of such a case.

Answers to Question 7

7.1 What is the abnormality seen in Figure 2.7.1?

Homogenous, lesion arising from the posterior third of the left vocal cord. This is most likely to represent a vocal cord granuloma. Vocal cord granulomas arise as a result of perichondritis of the cartilaginous vocal process of the arytenoids. This is thought to arise following repeated trauma to the overlying mucosa with resultant perichondrial inflammation. Trauma includes acid reflux, voice abuse, persistent coughing, and intubation.

7.2 Give the differential diagnosis.

Squamous cell cancer needs to be excluded by histological examination. Other differentials include papilloma, vocal cord polyp, vocal cord cyst, tuberculosis.

7.3 Give an account of the management of such a case.

Management depends on the severity of symptoms, the underlying cause and size of lesion and may require a combination of therapeutic strategies. Granulomas are notoriously difficult to treat and often recur since surgical excision will inevitably lead to further trauma to the area and more cartilage exposure.

- *History—important points:*
  - ◆ *Symptoms*—hoarseness, constant throat clearing, deep-seated sore throat, feeling of a lump in the throat, coughing following URTI
  - ◆ Occupation/voice abuse
  - ◆ Sergeant major, auctioneer, factory worker
  - ◆ Previous intubation—traumatic/prolonged in intensive care unit (ITU)
  - ◆ Laryngo-pharyngeal reflux
  - ◆ Smoking increases the possibility of a malignancy
- *Examination:*
  - ◆ Nasendoscopy
  - ◆ Oral cavity
  - ◆ Neck
- Treatment.

All patients require a microlaryngoscopy and biopsy to exclude squamous cell carcinoma (SCC). Excision of lesion may be performed by cold steel microsurgery or laser. Laser may result in a thermal insult to the tissues causing further chondritis of the arytenoid. Micro-rotation flaps have been used to cover the raw area of perichondrium following excision of the granuloma. Voice therapy may be used pre- and post-surgery, in combination with treatment of reflux even in the absence of classical reflux symptoms. Botulinum toxin has been used to temporarily paralyse the vocal cord to aid healing in patients where voice abuse seems the major etiological factor; this still remains somewhat controversial due to the increased risk of aspiration. Some advocate the use of steroids either intra-lesional, oral, or inhaled for recurrent granulomas.

Question 8

Figure 2.8.1 demonstrates a patient who is at risk of suffering a carotid blowout.

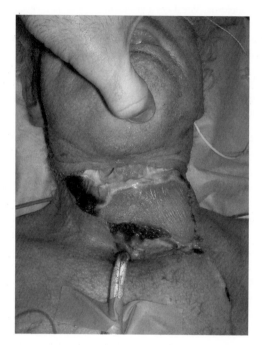

Figure 2.8.1 Patient at risk of suffering a carotid blowout.

8.1 What are the risk factors for this condition?

8.2 Describe the surgical steps you would take to prevent this complication during neck dissection.

8.3 How would you manage a patient who is at risk of this complication?

Answers to Question 8

8.1 What are the risk factors for this condition?

Spontaneous rupture of the carotid artery is a result of necrosis of the arterial wall.

Risk factors

Infection, poor nutrition, tumour invasion, previously irradiation. The risk has been found to be greatest when the radiation was given more than 6 months previously.

The commonest presentation is following a salvage (post-radiotherapy) surgical procedure with excision of primary tumour and neck dissection in which a post-operative salivary fistula develops adjacent to the carotid artery. Tumour dissection which necessitates removal of the adventitia of the artery devascularizes the vessel and predisposes to rupture.

The incidence of carotid blowout in patients following neck dissection regardless of whether the tumour has been resected has been reported as high as 3 to 4%. The presence of tumour around the carotid artery especially after radiotherapy and surgery increases this risk even further.

8.2 Describe the surgical steps you would take to prevent this complication during neck dissection.

Meticulous attention to pre-operative planning and operative technique is essential. Carefully placed skin incisions and the use of muscle flaps to cover the great vessels are the mainstays of prevention.

The site where three points in an incision meet is recognized as prone to poor healing and wound breakdown. Therefore in a previously irradiated neck one should avoid placing such a trifurcation over/close to the carotid sheath, classically this would involve a MacFee incision, but many surgeons find this awkward and prefer a lateral-T incision, which offers good access and the site where points of the incision meet lies posteriorly, and away from the carotid artery.

The major neck vessels can be protected by covering them with a muscle flap specifically raised for this purpose. A pectoralis major muscle only flap is most robust, but a local levator scapulae rotation flap can be mobilized by transecting it near its scapular insertion, and swinging it upwards to cover the vessel segment considered to be at greatest risk.

Vessels may also be protected by the same myocutaneous flap being used to reconstruct the post-excisional defect. This is particularly the case with a pedicled flap, e.g. pectoralis major compared free flaps, such as a radial forearm flap. When considering the reconstructive options for the surgical defect, the presence of a previously irradiated neck should be regarded as a significant factor in favour of using a pedicled myocutaneous flap, because of this incidental protective capacity.

8.3 How would you manage a patient who is at risk of this complication?

See Table 2.8.1.

Palliative	Curative	
	No bleeding	**Bleeding**
In the palliative setting treatment may be largely supportive and the patient should be advised of what may occur. Regular sedation and diamorphine should be prescribed in case of a catastrophic bleed. The patient's family should be counselled.	In the scenario where there is no history of bleeding, but with significant carotid artery exposure in an infected, fistulous and/or irradiated neck wound treatment should be directed towards developing an urgent plan for surgical debridement, repair of the fistula and carotid coverage with vascularized tissue, e.g. pectoralis major flap.	The appearance of anything that could be construed as slough of the vessel wall or the development of thrombosis of the vasa vasorum are evidence of impending rupture. Rupture rarely occurs unheralded; in the 48h before rupture there is usually a small prodromal bleed and this must be respected. The following steps should be taken: • Airway protected with a cuffed tracheostomy tube • Secure IV access • Cross-match 4U blood • Where exposed the artery should be covered by moist soaks. In the event of massive rupture ward staff should be instructed as follows: • Control bleeding with immediate finger pressure • Secure airway by inflating cuff on tracheostomy tube • Transfuse blood immediately.
		Interventional radiology available ⎮ **Interventional radiology not available** If this is available and patient is fit: Consider angiography + stenting/embolization ⎮ If not available or inappropriate then surgical intervention is only recourse.

Table 2.8.1

Further reading

Cohen J, Rad I (2004). Contemporary management of carotid blowout. *Curr Opin Otolaryngol Head Neck Surg* **12:** 110–15.

McGregor IA, Howard DJ (Eds). (1992). *Rob and Smith's Operative Surgery. Head and Neck*, Parts 1 and 2, 4th edn. Oxford: Butterworth–Heinemann.

Scott-Brown WG (1997). *Scott-Brown's Otolaryngology*, Vol. 5. Oxford: Butterworth-Heinemann.

Watkinson J, Gilbert RW (2012). *Stell and Maran's Textbook of Head and Neck Surgery and Onocology*, 5th edn. London: Hodder & Stoughton.

Question 9

9.1 Describe Figures 2.9.1 and 2.9.2 and give the diagnosis.

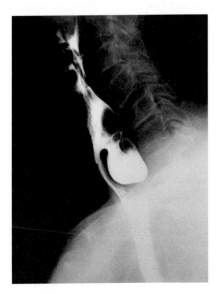

Figure 2.9.1

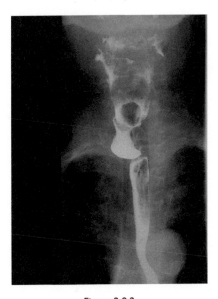

Figure 2.9.2

9.2 What are the classical presenting features of this condition?

9.3 What is the underlying aetiology?

9.4 Briefly describe the different modes of treatment in this condition.

9.5 Give a detailed surgical account of the open procedure.

Answers to Question 9

9.1 Describe Figures 2.9.1 and 2.9.2 and give the diagnosis.

These are lateral and AP radiographs of the neck with radio-opaque contrast (barium or possibly Gastrograffin), respectively.

They reveal the fundus of a pouch containing the radio-opaque contrast. The diagnosis is most likely a **pharyngeal pouch** (a posterior pharyngeal pulsion diverticulum, or Zenker's diverticulum).

9.2 What are the classical presenting features of this condition?

Symptoms

- Food sticking in throat
- Progressive dysphagia
- Regurgitation of undigested food, exacerbated by positional change, especially lying in bed at night.

This may wake patient at night when spillage from the pouch causes coughing and choking.

- Halitosis
- Gurgling noises emanating from the neck
- Swelling in the neck (nearly always on the left side).
- Weight loss
- Recurrent pneumonia due to aspiration
- Hoarseness, secondary to irritation of the VCs from repeated aspiration (or rarely because of involvement of the recurrent laryngeal nerve by a SCC arising in the pouch).

Signs

- Emaciation
- A soft swelling usually in the left lower part of the anterior triangle
- Swelling gurgles on palpation (Boyce's sign)
- A spasm of coughing may be caused by palpation due to spillage of contents into the larynx
- *Flexible nasendoscopy (FNE)*—demonstrates laryngitis and pooling of saliva in the pyriform fossa in which undigested food particles may be seen
- Rarely, blood may be found in the regurgitated contents of a pouch, suggesting development of a SCC of the pouch.

9.3 What is the underlying aetiology?

Pharyngeal pouches arise posteriorly by herniation of the pharyngeal mucosa through a relatively unsupported part of the posterior pharyngeal wall—the Killian's dehiscence. Mainly in men > 50 year old. Killian's dehiscence is a weak area at the lower part of the inferior constrictor muscle and is bounded by the two heads of the muscle, namely its cricopharyngeal and thyropharyngeal components. The cause is unknown, but pathogenesis probably multifactorial.

The most widely accepted theory is a pulsion diverticulum secondary to cricopharyngeal spasm, causing high intrapharyngeal pressure (Negus, 1950). While the cause of the spasm is unknown, poor coordination of swallowing may play a part. Once a pouch is formed, food enters it and stretches it even more so that it enlarges. It may remain static for many years or slowly increase in size until it eventually passes into the posterior mediastinum. Pressure from the pouch may then be exerted on the oesophagus from behind to cause dysphagia.

9.4 Briefly describe the different modes of treatment in this condition.

No treatment

This may be appropriate where the patient has few symptoms, is very old and infirm or in poor general condition.

Surgical options

- Endoscopic dilatation of the cricopharyngeal sphincter with bougies
  - ◆ Only temporary relief of symptoms
  - ◆ Does not remove the diverticulum generally leads to recurrence of symptoms
  - ◆ Risk of perforation
- Endoscopic division is generally regarded as the treatment of choice
  - ◆ Good results, low morbidity, and short hospital stay
  - ◆ Use of specialized endoscope with split beak
  - ◆ Endoscopic division of the bar between the pouch and the oesophagus
  - ◆ By dividing the party wall and cricopharyngeus using endoscopic staple gun (divide and staple synchronously). This division and widening the mouth of the diverticulum, it relieves the symptoms and restores swallowing
- *Open procedure*—the pouch may be excised, inverted or suspended via an external approach.

9.5 Give a detailed surgical account of the open procedure.

Diverticulectomy (excision of pouch)

- Once anaesthetized, oesophagoscopy is performed to confirm the diagnosis and exclude a synchronous carcinoma
- The pouch is packed with ribbon gauze in order to aid identification in the neck later in the procedure
- A bougie or anaesthetic ET tube is then placed into the oesophagus to facilitate the cricopharyngeal myotomy later in the procedure
- The patient is placed in a reverse Trendelenberg position with a sandbag under the shoulders and the head is extended and rotated away from the side of the incision
- A collar incision (usually on the left side of neck) is marked out on the skin at the level of the upper border of the cricoid from the midline to halfway across the sternocliedomastoid muscle, preferably in a skin crease
- The incision line is infiltrated with adrenaline to minimize bleeding and the incision made through skin, subcutaneous tissues, and platysma. Subplatysmal flaps are raised to demonstrate the strap muscles and sternocleidomastoid
- The deep cervical fascia is then incised along the anterior border of the sternocleidomastoid muscle, which is retracted laterally
- The omohyoid is identified, mobilized, and divided at which point the internal jugular vein comes into view
- The middle thyroid vein is divided and ligated so that the dissection may proceed medial to the carotid sheath, which is retracted laterally avoiding undue pressure on the carotid artery
- The inferior thyroid artery is identified and divided as necessary and if possible, the recurrent laryngeal nerve is identified at this point of the operation
- The packed diverticulum, can be easily identified by palpation and the fundus grasped with a pair of Babcock forceps
- The diverticulum is dissected free of the oesophagus, the thyroid gland and thyroid cartilage being retracted medially, with care not to damage the recurrent laryngeal nerve

- The neck of the pouch is then carefully cleaned of muscle fibres to its junction with the pharynx, which is identified by palpating the NGT
- Great care taken to avoid tearing the neck of the sac at this juncture
- The ribbon gauze pack is removed and stay sutures are inserted into the neck of the pouch inferiorly and superiorly, care being taken not to place them too medially, which would lead to a stricture
- The wound inferior to the neck of the pouch is packed with gauze to catch any debris, which may discharge and the pouch is amputated and sent to histology
- The mouth of the neck is closed with a continuous inverting suture and the stay sutures removed. A second layer of interrupted is used to bury the first
- The cricopharyngeal sphincter and upper circular fibres of the oesophagus are then displayed, stretched over the oesophageal bougie/endotracheal (ET) tube. The muscle fibres are divided avoiding damage to the recurrent laryngeal nerve
- Haemostasis is secured, a drain is inserted inferiorly, and the wound is closed in 2 layers
- Some surgeons use a stapling gun rather than performing a hand sewn pharyngeal repair
- An NGT is inserted under direct view and NG feeding is continued for 5–7 days, after which fluids are given
- If there are no complications, and the patient passes their post-operative contrast swallow the NGT is removed and a soft diet commenced.

Potential complications

- *Immediate:*
  - Primary haemorrhage
  - Surgical emphysema (mucosal tear or incomplete suture line)
- *Intermediate:*
  - Secondary haemorrhage (infection)
  - Hoarseness (recurrent laryngeal nerve damage)
  - Wound infection
  - Fistula (usually the result of infection)
  - Mediastinitis (leak tracking downwards)
- *Late:*
  - Persistent hoarseness (recurrent laryngeal nerve divided)
  - Stricture (too much mucosa excised when dividing the neck of the sac)
  - Recurrence (endoscopic diathermy 7%, diverticulectomy 2–3%).

Further reading

Bowdler DA (1997). Pharyngeal pouches. In Hibbert J (Ed.), *Scott-Brown's Otolaryngology*, Vol 5, 6th edn. London: Butterworth-Heinemann, Chapter 10.

Corbridge RJ (1998). The oesophagus and dysphagia. In *Essential ENT Practice—A Clinical Text*. London: Arnold (a member of the Hodder Headline Group), Chapter 6.

Negus VE (1950). Pharyngeal diverticula; observations on their evolution and treatment. *Br J Surg* **38**(150):129–46.

Roland NJ, McRae RD, and McCombe AW (2001). Pharyngeal pouch. In *Key Topics in Otolaryngology*, 2nd edn. BIOS Scientific Publishers Limited.

Question 10

10.1 Describe Figure 2.10.1.

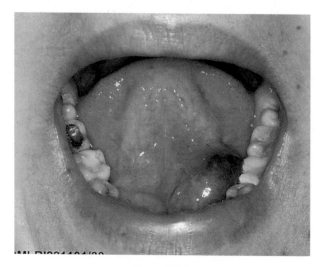

Figure 2.10.1

10.2 What is the diagnosis?

10.3 Are any investigations required?

10.4 Describe the underlying pathology.

10.5 Describe the management of such a case and what modifications you would make if this extended to the neck.

Answers to Question 10

10.1 Describe Figure 2.10.1.

The figure shows the oral cavity of an adult with a unilateral left sided sublingual dome shaped mass with intact epithelium. There is no displacement of the tongue. The mass is approximately 3 × 2cm and there is no evidence of a punctum or draining sinus.

10.2 What is the diagnosis?

A ranula. This will usually be diagnosed on clinical grounds alone; transillumination and bimanual palpation are helpful.

Differential diagnosis include:

- Benign or malignant salivary gland neoplasm
- Dermoid cyst
- Haemangioma
- Lymphangioma
- Soft tissue abscess.

10.3 Are any investigations required?

Usually not, but if there is any diagnostic uncertainty an MRI will be diagnostic

10.4 Describe the underlying pathology.

The development of a ranula depends on the disruption of the flow of saliva from the secretory apparatus of the salivary gland. Extravasation of mucus into the adjacent soft tissues forms a pseudocyst. This is most commonly initiated by a traumatic insult to the duct, but may also be due to partial or complete excretory duct obstruction. Causes include a sialolith, congenital malformation, stenosis, periductal fibrosis, or scarring from previous trauma, excretory duct agenesis, or tumour.

Most oral ranulas originate from the subligual gland and present in the tissues of the floor of the mouth. Should the pseudocyst extend inferiorly to the mylohyoid muscle, the ranula is called 'plunging' or cervical and may present as a diffuse level 1 neck lump.

10.5 Describe the management of such a case and what modifications you would make if this extended to the neck.

The management of oral ranulas may be conservative or surgical.

The traditional method is complete excision of the ranula and the associated major salivary gland.

An intra-oral excision of the sublingual gland is performed and lacrimal probe is inserted into the submandibular gland duct to aid its identification and dissection. The distal portion of this duct along with the attached sublingual gland is excised. Care must be taken to avoid damage to the lingual nerve. The remains of the submandibular duct are laid open and sutured to the floor of the mouth.

There is some evidence that marsupialization of the ranula with packing of the pseudocyst with gauze for a period of 7–10 days is as effective as complete excision. The entire ranula is unroofed and the subsequent packing of the cavity results in a foreign body reaction, sealing of the mucinous leak and allows for re- epithelialization to take place. Laser ablation and cryosurgery, either alone or with marsupialization, have also been used.

Recurrence rates of oral ranula with various treatments are quoted as:

- Incision and drainage 71–100%
- Excision only 0–25%
- Marsupialization 36–61%
- Marsupialization with packing 0%
- Excision ranula and salivary gland 0%.

The management of the cervical or 'plunging' ranula involves the complete excision of the oral part of the ranula and the associated sublingual salivary gland (or rarely the submandibular gland). The cervical ranula usually resolves and has a very low rate of recurrence. The most important aspect in the treatment of the plunging ranula is the excision of the responsible salivary gland.

Recurrence rates of cervical ranula with various treatments:

- Drainage cervical ranula alone 85%
- Gland excision intra-orally 0%
- Gland excision cervical approach 4%.

Question 11

This 38-year-old female presents with a snoring and a slowly enlarging lesion as shown in Figure 2.11.1.

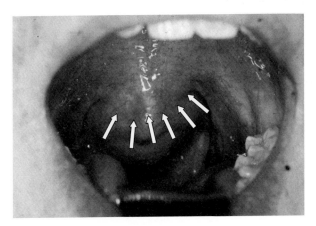

Figure 2.11.1

11.1 What is the differential diagnosis?

11.2 How would you proceed?

11.3 Your investigations suggest that this is a pleomorphic adenoma; what are the issues surrounding this patient's further management?

11.4 What would you recommend?

Answers to Question 11

11.1 What is the differential diagnosis?

See Table 2.11.1.

Lesions of the soft palate			Lesions of the PNS
Benign	Malignant	Others	Antrochoanal polyp
Pleomorphic adenoma	Adenoid cystic carcinoma	Cysts	Inflammatory polyps
Oxophilic adenoma	Mucoepidermoid	Granulomatous Diseases	Angiofibroma (in adolescent boy)
Fibroepithelioma	Acinic cell carcinoma		PNS neoplasms
Lipoma	Squamous cell carcinoma		Thornwalds cyst
Myoepithelial adenoma	Lymphoma		Craniopharyngioma
Osteoma			Chordoma

Table 2.11.1

11.2 How would you proceed?

Examination

Inspect position, size, pigmentation, ulceration.
- *Palpate*—hard or soft? Fixation to adjacent tissues, smooth or irregular, tender?
- *Nasendosopy*—looking for distortion of the floor of nose/superior surface of the soft palate, post-nasal space (PNS)
- Examination of neck and rest of aero-digestive tract.

Investigations

Tissue pathology is key: FNA if soft/Incisional Biopsy.
- *MRI*—will define the extent of the lesion and assess any nodal involvement
- CT may be required if there is any suggestion of hard palate involvement—bony erosion.

11.3 Your investigations suggest that this is a pleomorphic adenoma; what are the issues surrounding this patient's further management?

It is a benign tumour, but will continue to enlarge.

There are two treatment options.

Radical excision and reconstruction with sensate free flap or pedicled flap

If radical excision is undertaken, it will result in a large soft palate defect which can be reconstructed, but will still be associated with significant morbidity in terms of speech and swallowing. A mandibulotomy may be required for access. A temporary tracheostomy and NG tube may also be necessary.

Enucleation

Enucleation is associated with less morbidity, but the lesion may be more likely to recur. More is known about pleomorphic adenoma of the parotid gland. Here there is a 20–30% recurrence rate if simple enucleation is performed. Revision surgery in the parotid region is also associated with a 50% risk of facial nerve damage therefore complete excision, taking a good margin of normal tissue is indicated. Clearly, there is no risk to the facial or other nerve in surgery for recurrence in the soft palate. In addition tumor surveillance is easy in the oral cavity. Post-operative radiotherapy to reduce risk of recurrence is also an option.

11.4 What would you recommend?

In a young patient, I would recommend enucleation with close follow-up.

Question 12

An elderly gentleman is referred by his GP with proptosis.

12.1 What is proptosis and what are its common causes?

He complains of unilateral nasal obstruction and bloody rhinorrhoea and examination shows mass filling the right nasal cavity. You take a biopsy and request some imaging. The scans are shown in Figures 2.12.1–3.

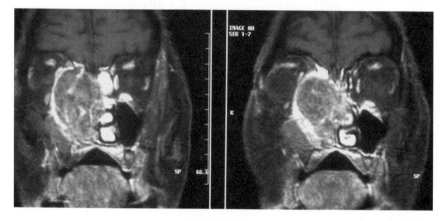

Figure 2.12.1

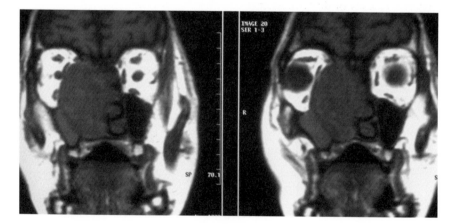

Figure 2.12.2

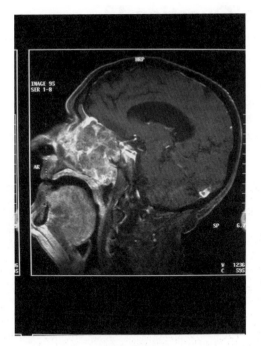

Figure 2.12.3

12.2 How would you interpret them?

12.3 Your biopsy shows adenocarcinoma; give a brief account of the aetiology and natural history of this condition

12.4 Discuss the management options in such a case.

Answers to Question 12

12.1 What is proptosis and what are its common causes?

Proptosis is unilateral protrusion of the orbit. In some texts, exophthalmos is used to describe proptosis due to endocrinological disorders.

Causes may be due to lesions either external to cone or within the cone—see Table 2.12.1.

External to cone	
Congenital:	Craniofacial abnormalities
Benign:	Frontal sinus mucocoele, osteoma
Malignant:	Tumour infiltration from ethmoid, sphenoid, or maxillary sinuses
	CNS, lymphoma, neuroblastoma (children)
Trauma:	Lateral trauma to the orbit
Infective:	Post-septal orbital cellulitis, pyocoeles
Within the cone	
Congenital:	Carotico-cavernous fistula
Benign:	Angioma, dermoid, meningioma or glioma of the optic nerve
Malignant:	Retinoblastoma, rhabdomyosarcoma, metastasis, e.g. melanoma
Inflammatory:	Thyroid eye disease
Trauma:	Retrobulbar haemorrhage

Table 2.12.1. Common causes of proptosis

12.2 How would you interpret Figures 2.12.1–3?

Shown are four coronal and one sagittal, T1-weighted MRI scans, the lower two are fat suppressed with contrast.

The obvious finding is destructive right-sided lesion in the nose and paranasal sinuses, crossing the midline, invading the right orbit, adjacent to, but not invading anterior cranial cavity extending posteriorly and extending to the post nasal space and sphenoid. The lesion looks malignant and the biopsy result is key to planning the future care of this patient.

12.3 Your biopsy shows adenocarcinoma; give a brief account of the aetiology and natural history of this condition.

The association of adenocarcinoma of the ethmoid sinuses and woodworking was first described by Macbeth in 1965 and later by Acheson in 1967. Miss E. Hadfield, a consultant ENT Surgeon at High Wycombe General Hospital, presented the first series of local furniture makers with the disease in 1970.

Hardwood dust is believed to contain large and small particles; the large particles interrupt mucocilliary clearance allowing longer surface exposure of the small (carcinogenic) particles to the sinonasal mucosa.

Typically, patients present up to 40 years after hardwood dust exposure. As in this case the typical symptoms are of unilateral nasal obstruction and associated bloody nasal discharge. The disease remains locally invasive, typically in the ethmoidal sinuses, and metastatic spread is rare. Destruction of bone and invasion of local structures is the usual cause of death. Aggressiveness of the disease varies depending on the histological grade of the tumour.

12.4 Discuss the management options in such a case.

These rare cancers must be managed in an MDT setting. Treatment is aimed at local control of the disease. Where possible primary surgery is preferred either via a cranio-facial resection or transantral ethmoidectomy. Post-operative external beam radiotherapy may be required however morbidity due to the effects of 'in field' local structures, especially the eye, may be considerable. An alternative therapy using topical 5-fluorouracil on nasal packs repeatedly applied to the surgical resection cavity has gained some popularity in mainland Europe (Knegt et al., 2001) where excellent results are claimed (see Further reading). Radiotherapy alone may be used as a primary modality for local control where the morbidity is expected to be less than that caused by an extensive surgical resection.

Further reading

Knegt PP, Ah-See KW, Velden LAV, Kerrebijn J (2001). Adenocarcinoma of the ethmoidal sinus complex: surgical debulking and topical fluorouracil may be the optimal treatment. *Arch Otolaryngol* **127**(2): 141–6.

Hadfield E (1989). Tumors of nose and sinuses in relation to wood workers. *J Laryngol* **33**: 417–22.

Ascheson EO, Hadfield EH, Macbeth RG (1967). Carcinoma of the nasal cavity and accessory sinuses in woodworkers. *Lancet* **1**: 311–12.

Macbeth R (1965). Malignant disease of the paranasal sinuses. *J Laryngol Otol* **79**: 592–612.

Question 13

13.1 Describe Figure 2.13.1 and the mode of action of the prosthesis.

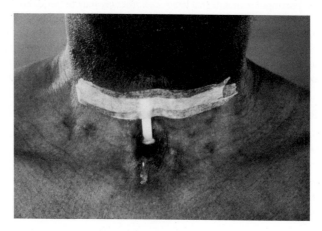

Figure 2.13.1

13.2 What are the important operative steps to consider when performing a total laryngectomy in order to achieve good voice rehabilitation?

13.3 If such a patient failed to achieve a good voice, how would you manage them?

Answers to Question 13

13.1 Describe Figure 2.13.1 and the mode of action of the prosthesis.

Clinical photo of laryngectomy patient with speaking valve—this is a Blom Singer 'ex-dwelling' variety. When the stoma is occluded these one way valves allow passage of air from the trachea into the vibrating pharyngo-oesophageal (PE) segment. This vibration creates noise and can be articulated through the mouth to produce voice. The valve also prevents leakage of oesophageal contents into the trachea.

13.2 What are the important operative steps to consider when performing a total laryngectomy in order to achieve good voice rehabilitation?

The PE segment should be capacious and pliable in order to allow sufficient vibration. In addition it should be sufficiently wide to give good swallowing. In order to give good post laryngectomy speech the surgical technique should include:

- An upper oesphageal myotomy
- A pharyngeal plexus neurectomy
- A tension free (and if possible) horizontal closure of the pharynx
- A primary puncture
- In addition division of the sternal heads of sterno-mastoid lead to a flattening of the lower neck which aids stomal dressing adhesion and humidity and moisture exchanger (HME) fixation.

13.3 If such a patient failed to achieve a good voice, how would you manage them?

- Consult your speech therapist to ensure good patient technique and optimal valve (e.g. if high pressure valve *in situ*, consider changing to low pressure valve)
- Check the valve patency and position, perform a nasedoscopy to check the internal positioning of the valve, if necessary remove the valve, allow the fistula tract to close and perform a staged secondary puncture
- If the problem seems to be due to the valve, try open tract speech and/or the Taube test
- If this fails to produce voice it suggests a problem with the PE segment, in which case check for recurrent tumour and PE segment stenosis under a general anaesthetic
- If there is no stenosis then consider video-fluoroscopy looking for PE spasm and if confirmed consider botox to the pharyngeal constrictor muscles/revision myotomy
- If all fails encourage oesophageal voice/electrical voice substitute.

Question 14

A 58-year-old solicitor presents with a 2-year history of discomfort in the left neck and localizes to the jugulodigastric region. The last doctor they saw in the clinic requested the investigations shown in Figure 2.14.1 and 2.14.2.

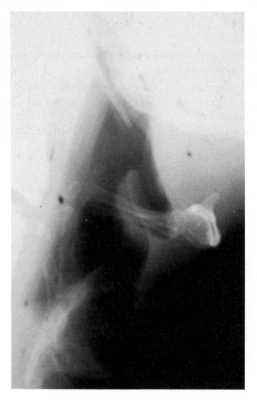

Figure 2.14.1

14.1 What is the likely diagnosis and aetiology?

14.2 What additional features would you like to demonstrate to confirm the diagnosis?

14.3 What is the 'definitive' diagnostic test?

14.4 Give a brief account of the surgical options in this case.

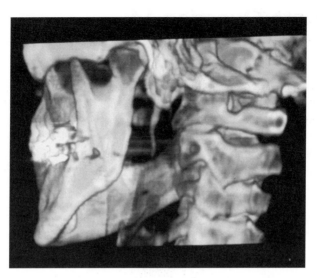

Figure 2.14.2

Answers to Question 14

14.1 What is the likely diagnosis and aetiology?

The most likely diagnosis is Eagle's syndrome. Eagle's syndrome occurs when an elongated styloid process or calcified stylohyoid ligament causes recurrent throat pain or foreign body sensation, dysphagia, or facial pain. Additional symptoms may include neck or throat pain with radiation to the ipsilateral ear.

Several pathophysiologic mechanisms leading to pain have been proposed:

(1) Traumatic fracture of the styloid process causing proliferation of granulation tissue, which may place pressure on the surrounding structures

(2) Compression of the adjacent nerves, the glossopharyngeal, lower branch of the trigeminal, or chorda tympani

(3) Degenerative and inflammatory changes in the tendinous portion of the stylohyoid insertion, called insertion tendinosis

(4) Irritation of the pharyngeal mucosa by direct compression or post-tonsillectomy scarring (involves cranial nerves V, VII, IX, and X)

(5) Impingement on the carotid vessels, producing irritation of the sympathetic nerves in the arterial sheath.

Marchetti (1652) first described the ossification of the stylohyoid ligament and there were several other isolated cases reported until Eagle described the syndrome in 1937.

Anatomy

The styloid process, stylohyoid ligament, and lesser cornu of the hyoid bone are derived from Reichert's cartilage, which arises from the second branchial arch. The cause of the elongation of the styloid process has not been fully elucidated. Proposed theories:
- Congenital elongation of the process due to persistence of a cartilaginous anlage in the stylohyale
- Calcification of the stylohyoid ligament giving the appearance of an elongated styloid process
- Growth of osseous tissue at the insertion of the stylohyoid ligament.

The styloid process is a slender, elongated, cylindrical bony projection that lies anteromedial to the mastoid process. It normally varies in length from 2–3cm. The styloid process has attachments to three muscles and two ligaments. The stylopharyngeus, stylohyoid, and styloglossus muscles originate here. The facial nerve emerges from the stylomastoid foramen posteriorly and passes laterally through the parotid gland. Medial to the styloid, moving posterior to anterior, are the internal jugular vein (with the XI, XII, X, and IX CN) and the internal carotid artery. Medial to the tip of the styloid process are the superior constrictor muscle and pharyngobasilar fascia, which lie adjacent to the tonsillar fossa. Lateral to the tip of the process is the external carotid artery, which bifurcates into the superficial temporal and maxillary arteries. The stylohyoid ligament extends from the styloid process to the lesser cornu of the hyoid bone.

14.2 What additional features would you like to demonstrate to confirm the diagnosis?

Diagnosis can usually be made on physical examination by digital palpation of the styloid process in the tonsillar fossa, which exacerbates the pain. There may also be loss of superficial temporal artery pulse on turning the head.

14.3 What is the 'definitive' diagnostic test?

Relief of symptoms with injection of a local anaesthetic solution into the tonsillar fossa is highly suggestive of this diagnosis.

14.4 Give a brief account of the surgical options in this case.

An intra-oral approach starts with an ipsilateral tonsillectomy after which the elongated styloid process will be easily palpable through the pharyngeal musculature (if this is not the case reconsider the diagnosis or the approach). The pharyngeal musculature is incised along the palpable bony abnormality. Using a Freer elevator the periosteum is stripped from the styloid and 2–3cm of the process can then be amputated using bone sheers or heavy scissors. The musculature can then be closed and the patient re-habilitated as per tonsillectomy guidelines.

In the external approach a 5cm horizontal skin incision is made 3–4cm below the mandibular ramus, at the anterior border of the sternocleidomastoid muscle. The deep cervical fascia is incised, and the anterior border of the sternocleidomastoid is retracted laterally. The stylohyoid muscle and the posterior belly of the digastric muscle are identified overlying the carotid arteries. The styloid process is exposed by retracting the muscles posteroinferiorly and the mandible anteriorly, carefully dissecting in the periosteal plane to the base of skull. The styloid process can then be shortened using bone-biting forceps. Careful dissection is required to avoid damage to the lower cranial nerves. A suction drain is usually placed and the wound closed in layers.

Further reading

Eagle WW (1937). Elongated styloid process: report of two cases. *Arch Otolaryngol* **25:** 584–6.

Marchetti D (1652). Anatomia. *Patavii* **13:** 205.

Question 15

A child presents with stridor.

15.1 Figure 2.15.1 is an endoscopic view of the larynx. Describe what you see.

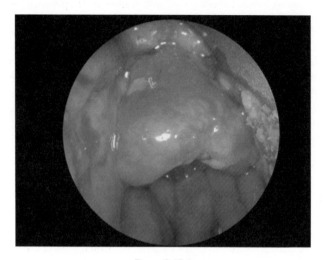

Figure 2.15.1

15.2 Give an account of the classical presentation of this condition.

15.3 Describe your management of such a case in A&E and in theatre.

15.4 Describe your technique in performing a tracheostomy in this case.

Answers to Question 15

15.1 Describe Figure 2.15.1

This is an endoscopic picture of a child with acute epiglottitis. The epiglottis would be expected to be cherry red and the aryepiglottic folds are grossly oedematous obliterating the view of the laryngeal inlet. This disease used to be caused most commonly by *Haemophilus influenza* type B (HIB), but since the HIB vaccine, other pathogens such as *Candida albicans*, *Haemophilus parainfluenza*, and *Staphylococcus* have become more common culprits. Nowadays this condition is most commonly seen in adults where there is a generalized inflammation of the entire supraglottis (supraglottitis).

15.2 Give an account of the classical presentation of this condition.

A child aged between 1–5 years presents with a history of an URTI that rapidly progresses to severe throat pain and dysphagia. Respiratory stridor then follows within hours. On examination, the child looks toxic (pale and shocked) and is drooling. He/she prefers to sit upright and lean forward. Speech is muffled if able to talk at all. There is usually marked cervical lymphadenopathy.

As the symptoms progress the child will become quiet, floppy and the respiratory rate will lessen. If no treatment is given extreme fatigue will lead to respiratory and cardiac arrest.

15.3 Describe your management of such a case in A&E and in theatre.

In A&E

Do not distress the child. The diagnosis is made on the history and limited signs at the foot of the bed. Allow the child to be comforted by parent who should hold him/her upright. Oxygen can be given. Contact most senior anaesthetist and ENT surgeon. Proceed directly to the operating room in order to secure airway.

In theatre

Make sure the following equipment is available: resuscitation trolley, naso- and oro-tracheal tubes ranging from 2.5mm upwards, laryngoscope, Storz ventilating bronchoscopes from 2.5 to 5mm and tracheostomy set.

- Breathe the child down with an inhalational technique in the upright position
- Muscle relaxants are avoided
- As soon as the child is asleep place him in supine or semi-prone position
- Anaesthesia is deepened to allow face mask ventilation and continuous positive airways pressure (CPAP)
- Avoid intubation too early as this may lead to laryngospasm
- Insert an intubating laryngoscope to confirm the diagnosis
- Swab epiglottis
- Make sure suction is available and switched on
- Aim the endotracheal tube at the anterior aspect of the laryngeal inlet with a semi-rigid introducer to displace the epiglottis anteriorly
- Then insert an appropriate oro-tracheal tube
- If initial attempts fail do not continue with repeated attempts as this will increase the oedema and can result in severe bradycardia and respiratory arrest
- If first intubation fails then use an age-appropriate, ventilating bronchoscope. If not available then use a Magills sucker to intubate the patient and allow adequate ventilation

- A bougie or suction catheter can then be inserted and used as a guide to placement an oral or nasal endotracheal tube
- Once the airway is established the tube is firmly secured. IV access is obtained and cefotaxime, chloramphenicol is given
- NGT is inserted to decompress the stomach. The child may then be safely transferred to paediatric intensive care unit (PICU)
- Extubate with steroid cover when there is evidence of a leak around the tube with airway pressure of 20cm of water.

If unable to intubate then proceed with tracheostomy.

15.4 Describe your technique in performing a tracheostomy in this case.

- It is preferable to perform tracheostomy with the bronchoscope in place. Check appropriate tracheostomy tubes are available
- Extend the neck and place a shoulder roll. (Do not hyperextend as mediastinal structures can come into the neck)
- Remove any oesphageal tubing
- *Identify thyroid and cricoid cartilages*—this can be difficult as they are very soft and located in a more superior position than in adults. Mark the anatomical landmarks
- *Perform an incision*—one finger breath above the suprasternal notch
- The midline fascia lifted and divided and straps retracted laterally
- Isthmus usually does not need to be divided
- The trachea is identified and stay sutures are placed 2mm from midline around at least two tracheal rings
- Make vertical trachea incision centred upon the 2–4th rings
- Insert tube by exerting traction on the stay sutures
- Secure tube with sutures and ties
- Post-operative humidified oxygen, suction, and CXR.

Question 16

You are seeing a 65-year-old lady who complains of weakness of the right side of her face. In the course of your examination, you note an area on her forehead consistent with previous cutaneous surgery and a skin graft. There is also a fullness in her right parotid.

16.1 What is the likely chain of events that led to this current condition?

16.2 How would you suggest this patient is further managed?

16.3 How would you manage the weakness of eye closure?

16.4 What are the options available regarding facial reanimation?

Answers to Question 16

16.1 What is the likely chain of events that led to this current condition?

It is likely that the patient has had a cutaneous malignancy (probably a squamous cell carcinoma) excised from forehead with skin graft. The patient now represents with metastatic deposits to the pre-auricular/intra- parotid lymph nodes gland. Malignant infiltration of the VIIth nerve has caused a lower motor neuron facial palsy.

16.2 How would you suggest this patient is further managed?

- FNA of the parotid mass to confirm diagnosis
- MRI neck looking for associated deep cervical nodes, CT chest/CXR to exclude distant metastases and stage the disease
- This patient's treatment depends on the stage of the disease, patient co-morbidities, and wishes and these discussions should occur within the context of an MDT
- If the patient is otherwise fit and the disease is limited to the neck, surgical treatment with post-operative radiotherapy gives this patient the best chance of cure. This would involve an extended radical parotidectomy, taking both superficial and deep lobes of the parotid, facial nerve and modified radical neck dissection.

16.3 How would you manage the weakness of eye closure?

Prophylactic eye care to protect against corneal desiccation should be instigated. This should as a minimum include eye tapes at night and artificial tears. At surgery consideration should be given to performing a tarsorraphy +/− a gold weight implant to aid eye closure.

16.4 What are the options available regarding facial reanimation?

Dynamic

Aims to restore tone and movement:

1 Direct anastomosis performing an epineural repair using a 9.0/10.0 monofilament suture
2 Inter-positional grafts can be used if there is a long nerve defect or the anastomosis is put under excessive tension
   (a) Sural nerve is found posterior to the lateral malleolus of the ankle, this gives a long graft (20–30cm), and can be split to allow more than one anastomosis
   (b) Greater auricular is found running over the surface of sternocleidomastoid. This is suitable for a short graft (3–4cm), allows only one anastomosis
3 Cross-over techniques: the most common of which is hypoglossal to facial anastomosis. This involves an inter-positional graft between the hypoglossal and facial nerves in order to preserve hypoglossal function. Other variations described include spinal accessory to facial, contralateral facial to ipsilateral facial. A cross-over facial nerve graft followed by a free muscle transfer graft may provide some dynamic function
4 Muscle transfer: pedicled muscle transposition, e.g. temporalis or masseter are most commonly used, but free muscle trasfer, e.g. gracilis, serratus anterior, extensor digitorum brevis may be considered.

Static

Aims to restore tone, but no movement.

1 In cases of complete facial paralysis, where due to the patients age or need for post-operative radiotherapy means that nerve grafting is unlikely to give a good result other static methods can be considered. Here, facial slings may be considered.

2 Facial plastic procedures may also be helpful, e.g. rhytidectomy, blepharoplasty and brow lift.

Question 17

A 64-year-old man presents with a lesion in his oral cavity. There are no palpable lymph nodes in the neck.

17.1 Describe the abnormality in Figures 2.17.1 and 2.17.2 of this patient.

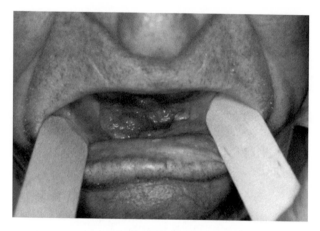

Figure 2.17.1

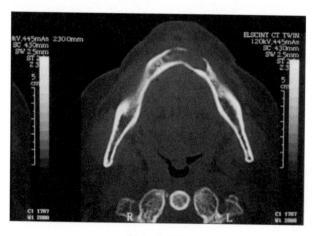

Figure 2.17.2

A biopsy confirms squamous cell carcinoma and his staging CT shows no obviously abnormal nodes and no distant metastatic spread. Prior to presenting this patient at the MDT your consultant suggests you discuss the possible treatment options.

17.2 What is the likely TNM staging is this patient?

17.3 Are there any other investigations that may be helpful in planning treatment?

17.4 Discuss the options and issues surrounding the treatment to the primary tumour and the neck.

17.5 How would you treat this patient?

Answers to Question 17

17.1 Describe the abnormality in Figures 2.17.1 and 2.17.2 of this patient

There is an exophytic and ulcerative irregular mass arising from the inferior alveolar margin in the midline. The axial CT at level of mandible shows a corresponding bony erosion of outer cortex.

17.2 What is the likely TNM staging is this patient?

In view of bony involvement: T4a N0 M0.

17.3 Are there any other investigations that may be helpful in planning treatment?

An orthopantomogram (OPG) to delineate the height of the mandible (which can be reduced if edentulous) and the site of the mental foramen may be helpful when planning a bony resection, i.e. marginal or segmental.

17.4 Discuss the options and issues surrounding the treatment to the primary tumour and the neck.

These patients must be discussed in an appropriate MDT and the decisions taken must reflect the patient's wishes and co-morbidities.

In general, treatment of the clinically/radiological N0 neck is recommended if the incidence of occult metastasis exceeds 15–20%. This is the case for most oral cavity cancers, with the exception of some small T1 tumours. Tumours involving the midline will usually require both sides of the neck to be treated.

The treatment of the neck will usually be determined by how the primary site is treated, with the aim of using the same modality to treat both sites. (The rationale for this is to maximize chance of cure whilst minimizing treatment associated morbidity).

Surgery is the mainstay for treating most oral cavity squamous cell carcinomas especially if bony involvement since this is poorly treated with radiotherapy. The main issues concerning surgery to this lesion include:

Access

Trans-oral would be appropriate if no bony reconstruction is required and local tissues are to be used to cover the defect. A visor incision would be required to give access to the neck if free flap surgery is required.

Resection of the mandible

Marginal/segmental that will depend upon the extent of involvement and height of the mandible. Periosteal involvement may require only a marginal resection; involvement of bone will require a segmental resection.

How to reconstruct the hard and soft tissue defects

If a marginal resection of the mandible is performed, the soft tissue defect may be closed with a local mucosal advancement flap or a distant soft tissue flap.

If a segmental resection of the anterior mandible is necessary, reconstruction will be required. Reconstruction of the mandible aims to restore contour, mastication (especially important with anterior mandibular defects), speech, lip and oral cavity sensation, and restoration of dentition.

Reconstruction options in this situation would include reconstruction plate with a soft tissue flap to cover such as a radial free forearm flap, or an osseous free flap, such as a fibula free flap (which has the advantage of good functional restoration with the possibility of osseointegrated implants, but this needs careful consideration in the irradiated mandible).

In patients where free flap reconstruction is required the major vessels in the neck will need to be exposed for anastamosis. A selective neck dissection adds little morbidity to the procedure and will be required to give vascular access. In addition if the neck is proven histologically to be node negative this may spare the patient the morbidity associated with bilateral neck irradiation.

Surgical treatment for the N0 neck will involve a selective neck dissection with removal of node levels most at risk.

In advanced oral cavity cancer (T3/4 N0 or T1–4 N+), surgery is usually followed by post-operative radiotherapy, and the neck may be spared if the nodal sampling from the bilateral selective neck dissection is negative.

If there are adverse features from the histology such as positive resection margins or nodal extra-capsular spread, then chemoradiotherapy should be considered.

NB: if a decision was made to treat the primary with radiotherapy, the N0 neck would also be treated with radiotherapy.

17.5 How would you treat this patient?

After discussion in the MDT and with the patient I would recommend surgical excision of the primary site with a free fibula flap reconstruction with skin to reconstruct the mucosal defect. In addition a bilateral level I–IV selective neck dissection to sample the nodes most at risk. Depending on the results of histology, the patient may also be offered post-operative radiotherapy.

Further reading

Head and Neck Cancer: Multidisciplinary Management Guidelines. ENT UK. September 2011. Available at: https://entuk.org/docs/prof/publications/head_and_neck_cancer

Question 18

18.1 See Figure 2.18.1. What procedure has been carried out here?

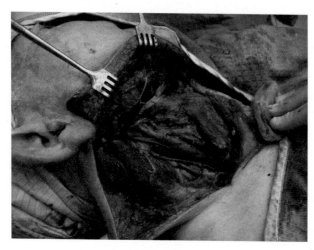

Figure 2.18.1

18.2 In the classical operation what structures are removed?

18.3 What are the indications for performing a complete neck dissection?

18.4 What are types 1, 2, and 3 modified radical neck dissection (RND)?

18.5 What is a functional neck dissection?

18.6 What is a selective neck dissection and when is it used?

Answers to Question 18

18.1 See Figure 2.18.1. What procedure has been carried out here?

A radical/complete neck dissection, clearing all 5 nodal levels.

18.2 In the classical operation what structures are removed?

All lymph-bearing tissue from mandible to clavicle, i.e. all five nodal groups, the sterno-mastoid muscle, internal jugular vein, accessory nerve, and submandibular gland.

18.3 What are the indications for performing a complete neck dissection?

The N positive neck. This is a traditional indication for level 1–5 nodal clearance. However there is an increasing practice of performing a selective neck dissection even in the presence of nodal disease.

18.4 What are types 1, 2, and 3 modified RND?

In all these types of neck dissection all 5 nodal levels are cleared as in a classical radical neck dissection. However, here the technique is modified in order to preserve certain structures:

- *Type 1*—preservation of spinal accessory nerve
- *Type 2*—preservation of spinal accessory nerve and internal jugular vein
- *Type 3*—preservation of spinal accessory nerve, internal jugular vein, and sternocleidomastoid.

18.5 What is a functional neck dissection?

The same as a modified radical neck type 3 dissection, i.e. preservation of function.

18.6 What is a selective neck dissection and when is it used?

Here, a less than complete nodal clearance is performed, i.e. nodal levels are dissected in accordance with the site of the primary tumour (see Box 18.1). It is best thought of as a lymph node sampling operation. In all cases it is performed for N0 neck disease. The choice of dissection is based on the risk of nodal metastases from that primary site.

- Supraomohyoid (levels I, II, and III) neck dissection performed for lip and oral cavity tumours
- Lateral (levels II, III, and IV) neck dissection performed for laryngeal and hypopharyngeal tumours
- Posterolateral (levels II, III, IV, and V) neck dissection for skin tumours of the scalp and occiput
- Anterior compartment (level VI, VII) neck dissection for thyroid cancer and some laryngeal cancers.

Box 2.18.1 **Boundaries of cervical lymph node groups**

I   Submental and submandibular triangles, area bounded by anterior belly digastric, hyoid, posterior belly digastric and the body of the mandible

II Upper 1/3 IJV, hyoid bone to skull base

III Middle 1/3 IJV, cricoid to hyoid bone

IV Lower 1/3 IJV, clavicle to cricoid

V   Posterior triangle, between posterior border of sternocleidomastoid (SCM) and anterior border trapezius including supraclavicular nodes

VI Pre- and paratracheal, hyoid to suprasternal notch

VII Superior mediastinum.

NB. Bifurcation of carotid is at the level of the hyoid bone at C4.

Question 19

This patient presents with hoarseness and the laryngeal appearances as shown in Figure 2.19.1

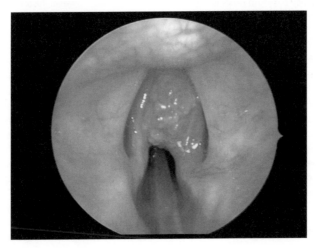

Figure 2.19.1

19.1 What is the likely diagnosis?

19.2 Give a brief account of this condition.

19.3 How could you manage this patient medically?

19.4 How would you treat this patient surgically?

Answers to Question 19

19.1 What is the likely diagnosis?

Recurrent respiratory papillomatosis is the most likely diagnosis; however histology will differentiate this from vocal cord granuloma and squamous cell carcinoma which could have similar appearances.

19.2 Give a brief account of this condition.

This condition is due to epithelial infection with HPV subtypes 6 or 11; the latter is associated with the more aggressive and troublesome disease. The laryngeal lesions often have a characteristic lobulated appearance and may be single or multifocal; histology confirms keratinizing squamous papillomas. The lesions commonly affect the free edges of mucosal surfaces in the upper aero-digestive tract, e.g. the uvula and soft palate, tonsil, and vocal fold. In the larynx they present with increasing hoarseness and when severe stridor. Rarely may they affect the entire respiratory tract including the tracheobronchial tree. The more aggressive lesions are most often seen in children than indults, with a peak incidence of between 2–5 years. Remission may occur spontaneously, but early onset and severe disease make it less likely. It is not associated with the onset of puberty, and relapse may be precipitated by trauma or immunosuppression.

19.3 How could you manage this patient medically?

Generally one should ensure good vocal technique and involve speech and language therapy.

Adjuvant therapies

- Indole—3-carbinol (an anti—oestrogen); Phase 1 trial in May 2013
- Interferon can be useful in severe cases and aids regression
- Photodynamic therapy (PDT)
- Intra-leisonal cidofovir has been shown to have some benefit although the response is not predictable.
- Avastin (bevacizumab) is a monoclonal antibody which shows promise as a therapeutic agent.

19.4 How would you treat this patient surgically?

Surgical excision with careful technique is essential. Care must be taken to avoid excessive damage to the free edge of the vocal fold and anterior commissure. Debate exists over the differing surgical tools of preference. Essentially this boils down to cold steel/micro-debridement vs. CO_2 laser (see Table 2.19.1).

Cold Steel	Laser
No thermal burn ∴ a reduced chance of scarring adverse voice outcome	Less blood loss
No vapour plume	Pinpoint accuracy. Vapour plume in which viral particles have been found and hence put the operator and theatre staff at some risk
Better tactile feedback	Improved access to difficult areas
Excellent for de-bulking of large papilloma deposits	Endotracheal fire risk

Table 2.19.1

Immuno-therapeutics and gene mapping may be useful adjuncts in the future.

Question 20

This patient presents to A&E with marked inspiratory stridor. Figure 2.20.1 shows laryngeal appearance during inspiration.

20.1 Describe and interpret the findings in Figures 2.20.1 and 2.20.2.

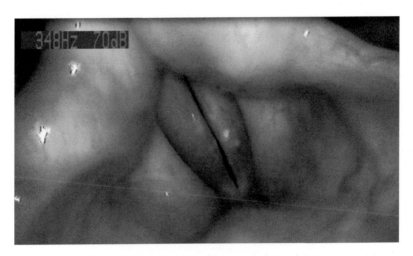

Figure 2.20.1 Laryngeal appearance during inspiration.

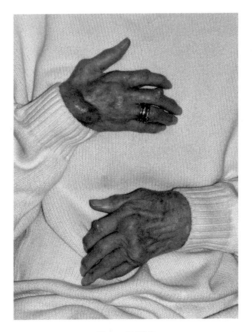

Figure 2.20.2

20.2 What are the issues related to the management of the airway in *this* case?

20.3 What are the options in managing the airway in this case? Describe the advantages and disadvantages of each.

Answers to Question 20

20.1 Describe and interpret the findings in Figures 2.20.1 and 2.20.2.

The patient has the classical hand signs seen in rheumatoid arthritis: rheumatoid nodules. The picture shows a static picture of the larynx, but as the patient is presenting with stridor it may be assumed that the picture represents a failure of abduction of the vocal cords resulting in a compromise of the airway at the glottis.

Main cause of inspiratory stridor in a patient with rheumatoid arthritis, with a non-inflamed larynx and with no obvious obstructive mass, is crico-arytenoid joint fixation secondary to rheumatoid changes in this synovial joint. Although not evident here, 'bamboo lesions' on vocal folds have been described corresponding to rheumatoid nodule-like deposits seen elsewhere in the body.

20.2 What are the issues related to the management of the airway in *this* case?

In the acute setting one may expect a relatively poor response to steroids and adrenaline as there is no mucosal inflammatory component and it is likely that the patient has a high steroid tolerance.

A difficult endotracheal intubation may be predicted due to poor joint mobility of the C-spine, temporo-mandibular joints, rigid fixed cords.

Tracheostomy may need to be performed under local anaesthetic. The patient will have poor manual dexterity and as a result managing a tracheostomy may be difficult for them. Any endoscopic procedure to alleviate the obstruction may prove difficult due to the limited access and may compromise both the voice of the patient and reduce the protection of the airway with possible aspiration thereafter.

20.3 What are the options in managing the airway in this case? Describe the advantages and disadvantages of each.

See Table 2.20.1.

Intervention	General	Airway	Voice	Aspiration Risk
Oral steroids	No operation Systemic side effects	Variable, Poor if joint is ankylosed	Good	None
Intra-joint steroids	Minor procedure May be poor access Not a long-term solution	Variable results. Poor result if joint is ankylosed	Good	None
Laser cordectomy/ arytenoidectomy	May be poor access Irreversible	Moderate	Poor	Moderate
Vocal cord lateralization procedure (e.g. suture abduction)	May be poor access, Unreliable result, Reversible	Good	Poor	Moderate
Tracheostomy	Poor dexterity = difficult to manage tracheostomy	Excellent	Good	Low

Table 2.20.1

Chapter 3

Otology

Question 1

1.1 Describe Figure 3.1.1. What is the likely diagnosis and what are the key findings on imaging that lead you to this diagnosis?

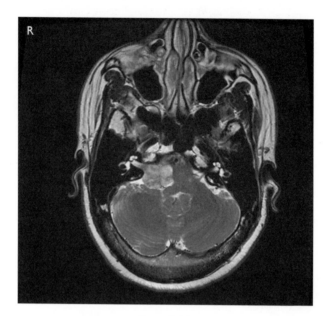

Figure 3.1.1

1.2 How might this patient present?

1.3 What would your examination comprise?

1.4 What are the other possible diagnoses for a lesion at this site?

1.5 Assuming the most likely diagnosis, how is this condition managed?

1.6 What are the different surgical approaches to treat this lesion and what are their relative advantages/disadvantages?

1.7 How might age affect the surgical approach used?

1.8 What are the potential complications of surgery?

Answers to Question 1

1.1 Describe Figure 3.1.1. What is the likely diagnosis and what are the key findings on imaging that lead you to this diagnosis?

Axial cut T2-weighted MRI at level of the cerebellopontine angle (CPA) showing mass filling right internal acoustic meatus (IAM) and extending into CPA with some minor compression of cerebellar peduncle, consistent with an acoustic neuroma/vestibular schwannoma.

1.2 How might this patient present?

Unilateral sensori-neural hearing loss (present in 95%), which may have a sudden deterioration in (10–20%), unilateral tinnitus (65%), disequilibrium common (50%), but vertigo uncommon (20%) due to slow growth allowing central compensation, facial paraesthesia (V), and facial nerve dysfunction (VII).

Large tumours may go on to cause diplopia, hoarseness, dysphagia, cerebellar symptoms, and signs of raised intracranial pressure such as headaches and vomiting.

1.3 What would your examination comprise?

Full neurotological examination to include trigeminal nerve sensation (corneal reflex), cerebellar signs, and ?paraesthesia of posterior auditory canal—Hitselberger sign.

1.4 What are the other possible diagnoses for a lesion at this site?

Includes: meningioma (differentiated from an acoustic neuroma (AN) by broad base, dural tail, and absence of IAM expansion), epidermoid, arachnoid cyst, lipoma, as well as lesions extending from skull base, such as glomus tumours, chordomas, and cholesterol granulomas.

1.5 Assuming the most likely diagnosis, how is this condition managed?

Observation with serial MRI scanning, surgery and radiotherapy (gamma knife/stereotactic radiotherapy).

1.6 What are the different surgical approaches to treat this lesion and what are their relative advantages/disadvantages?

Translabyrinthine

Pros: good access for most tumours especially lateral IAM involvement, minimal retraction of the brain and avoidance of problems related to this, wide exposure to CPA, highest facial nerve preservation rates.
Cons: complete loss of hearing, short-term vertigo if residual vestibular function pre-operatively.

Retrosigmoid

Pros: good for tumours with serviceable hearing as hearing preservation possible (30–65%), wide exposure CPA, and good facial nerve preservation rate.
Cons: fundus not visualized; therefore, not appropriate for tumours involving lateral IAM, cerebellar retraction, persistent post-operative headache in 10%.

Middle fossa

Pros: good for small <1cm intracanalicular tumours with limited involvement of CPA, high rates of hearing preservation, reduced risk of CSF leak.

Cons: technically most difficult due to lack of surgical landmarks/narrow access/unfavourable position of facial nerve during dissection. Temporal lobe retraction with risk of epilepsy requiring 1 year of anticonvulsant therapy and cessation of driving during this time.

1.7 How might age affect the surgical approach used?

In the older population, cerebral/cerebellar atrophy improves the access through a retrosigmoid approach, reducing the need for cerebellar retraction meaning this approach may be favoured. In addition, the dura may be more adherent and fragile in this group making the middle fossa approach less favourable.

1.8 What are the potential complications of surgery?

Facial weakness, hearing loss, intracranial haemorrhage/stroke, CSF leak (10–15%), syndrome of inappropriate anti-diuretic hormone secretion (SIADH), meningitis, death (1%).

Question 2

A 75-year-old lady presents to clinic with hearing loss in the left ear. Following removal of wax and crust from the left ear, the image shown in Figure 3.2.1 is obtained with a 0 degree endoscope.

2.1 Describe Figure 3.2.1.

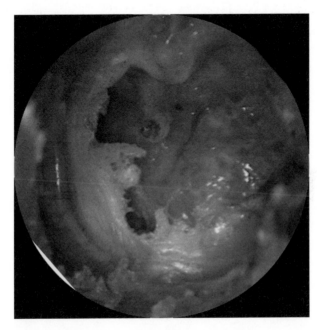

Figure 3.2.1

2.2 Please identify some anatomical structures.

2.3 What details would be important in the history in this patient and why?

2.4 How would you manage this patient?

2.5 What factors may predispose to a persistently discharging mastoid cavity?

2.6 What is a tympanic neurectomy and when is it performed?

Answers to Question 2

2.1 Describe Figure 3.2.1.

- Very abnormal
- Subtotal perforation of tympanic membrane (TM) with irregular edge and keratin/cholesteatoma medial to TM in anteroinferior quadrant at least
- Posteroinferior retraction of TM onto promontory
- Handle of malleus, long process of incus and stapes suprastructure all eroded.

2.2 Please identify some anatomical structures.

See Figure 3.2.2.

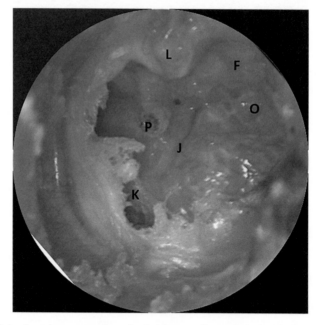

Figure 3.2.2 L—lateral process malleus; F—facial nerve; O—oval window; J—Jacobsen's nerve; P—processus cochleariformis; K—keratin.

2.3 What details would be important in the history in this patient and why?

Symptoms from ear

- Otorrhoea, tinnitus, vertigo, and timescale of onset of hearing loss
- State of contralateral ear including hearing
- Medical comorbidities
- Anaesthetic risk.

2.4 How would you manage this patient?

If medically fit and problematic otorrhoea, could consider tympanomastoid surgery probably in the form of single stage modified radical mastoidectomy. However, in view of her age and minimal symptoms, this lady would be best managed conservatively with regular aural toilet in outpatients department (OPD).

2.5 What factors may predispose to a persistently discharging mastoid cavity?

- Inadequate meatoplasty
- High facial ridge
- Uneven cavity/inadequate saucerization
- Residual cholesteatoma
- Perforation in neotympanum
- Large cavity/sump.

2.6 What is a tympanic neurectomy and when is it performed?

Division of Jacobsen's nerve to treat Frey's syndrome.

Figure 3.2.2 shows an annotated diagram.

Question 3

A 32-year-old female patient presents to clinic with a 3-year history of hearing loss in the right ear. Otoscopy is normal.

3.1   What does the audiogram show (Figures 3.3.1 and 3.3.2)? What further information would you want?

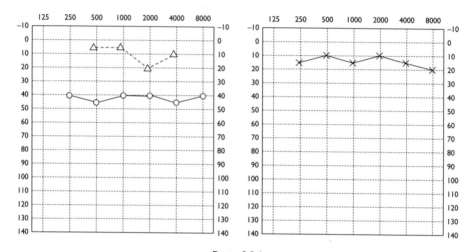

Figure 3.3.1

3.2   What is Carhart's notch?

3.3   What does the tympanogram measure and how can the results be classified?

3.4   For this patient, what are the main differential diagnoses?

3.5   What information in the history would help decide on the most likely diagnosis?

3.6   What is paracusis Willisii?

3.7   What would be your initial management?

3.8   When considering a patient for stapedectomy, what additional tests may be helpful?

3.9   When consenting a patient for stapes surgery, of which risks would you warn them?

3.10   What are the relative and absolute contraindications to stapes surgery?

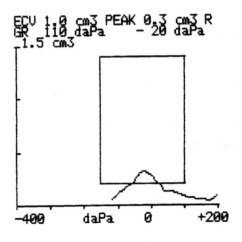

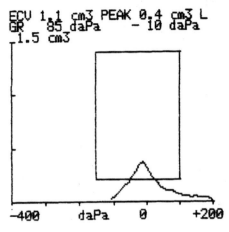

Figure 3.3.2

Answers to Question 3

3.1 What does the audiogram show (Figures 3.3.1 and 3.3.2)? What further information would you want?

This audiogram shows normal hearing on the left with hearing loss on the right with air conduction (AC) thresholds between 40 and 50dB. The unmasked bone conduction thresholds are around 10dB showing good cochlear reserve with a dip at 2kHz (Carhart's notch). Masked bone conduction thresholds are required to determine if this is truly a conductive loss.

3.2 What is Carhart's notch?

Carthart's notch is an artefactual dip in bone conduction (BC)/cochlear threshold at 2KHz seen in conductive hearing loss, which resolves/improves on correction of the conductive defect.

The cause for this is debated, but may be explained as follows. When attempting to test only cochlear function with BC thresholds, some of the sound inadvertently also travels via the tympanic membrane and ossicles to the inner ear. The natural resonance frequency of the ear canal/TM/middle ear/ ossicles is around 2KHz meaning this effect is greatest at this frequency. Therefore, if a conductive hearing loss occurs, this will inadvertently also reduce the apparent BC threshold across all frequencies but most markedly at 2KHz.

3.3 What does the tympanogram measure and how can the results be classified?

Tympanometry is a measure of tympanic membrane compliance (admittance), which is inversely related to acoustic impedance (the resistance to the passage of sound energy). Compliance is maximal when the external canal pressure is equal to the middle ear pressure. Type A, B, C1, C2.

3.4 For this patient, what are the main differential diagnoses?

- Otosclerosis
- Ossicular chain discontinuity/fixation
- Tympanosclerosis
- Cholesteatoma.

3.5 What information in the history would help decide on the most likely diagnosis?

- History of ear infections/trauma/previous surgery
- Progression (pregnancy)
- Family history of conductive hearing loss/otosclerosis.

3.6 What is paracusis Willisii?

Improved hearing (of speech) in the presence of background noise.

3.7 What would be your initial management?

Hearing aid trial for at least 6 months. (Discuss future hearing loss associated with pregnancy.)

3.8 When considering a patient for stapedectomy, what additional tests may be helpful?

Tuning fork tests

If Rinne negative (BC>AC) with 512Hz and 1024Hz, there is a high probability that the air-bone gap is sufficiently large for the patient to have a good outcome from stapes surgery.

Speech audiometry

If speech discrimination <60%, the patient may have cochlear otosclerosis and would be a poor candidate for surgery.

3.9 When consenting a patient for stapes surgery, of which risks would you warn them?

Dead ear (0.5–1%), floating or depressed footplate, incomplete closure of A–B gap (5%), altered taste, vertigo, tinnitus, facial nerve palsy, abandon procedure (due to persistent stapedial artery, overhanging facial nerve, wrong diagnosis), reparative granuloma, late failure.

3.10 What are the relative and absolute contraindications to stapes surgery?

Relative contraindications

- Only hearing ear
- Severe vertigo after first stapedectomy
- Poor speech discrimination (<60%)
- Mixed loss where they will still need to wear hearing aid after surgery
- Patients with preoperative vertigo.

Absolute contraindications

Active external or middle ear infection.

Question 4

4.1 What proportion of congenital hearing loss is genetic?

4.2 What proportion of these are syndromic/non-syndromic?

4.3 What is the commonest genetic abnormality causing non-syndromic hearing loss?

4.4 Give 3 examples of the more common syndromic causes of (sensorineural) hearing loss with their characteristics?

4.5 How can we test a child's hearing and at what age can these tests be performed?

4.6 What investigations would you perform on an otherwise normal baby with audiologically confirmed profound bilateral hearing loss? Please briefly state the rationale for each investigation.

4.7 What is the benefit of investigating for an aetiology?

Answers to Question 4

4.1 What proportion of congenital hearing loss is genetic?

50%.

4.2 What proportion of these are syndromic/non-syndromic?

Of the genetic hearing loss: 1/3 syndromic, 2/3 non-syndromic.

4.3 What is the commonest genetic abnormality causing non-syndromic hearing loss?

Mutations in the gap junction beta 2 (*GJB2*) gene, which encodes the protein connexin-26, accounts for 50% of autosomal recessive non-syndromic hearing loss.

Connexin 26 is a gap junction protein expressed in sites, such as the stria vascularis and basement membrane, and is responsible for the intercellular transport of ions. It is thought to be involved in replenishing the potassium ions back into the endolymph after stimulation of the sensory hair cells.

4.4 Give 3 examples of the more common syndromic causes of (sensorineural) hearing loss with their characteristics?

- *Pendred's syndrome*—progressive sensorineural hearing loss (SNHL), goitre, which may not be evident until late childhood, hypothyroid/euthyroid, widened vestibular aqueduct, Mondini malformation
- *Usher's syndrome*—SNHL with progressive loss of vision due to retinitis pigmentosa
- *Waardenburg syndrome*—SNHL with white forelock, wide confluent eyebrows, dystopia canthorum, premature graying of hair/eyelashes/eyebrows, heterochromia irides/sapphire eyes. May be associated with Hirschprungs, hypoplastic limbs
- *Alport syndrome*—SNHL often high tone, glomerulonephritis with haematuria progressing to renal failure, retinal flecks. Defective type 4 collagen causes abnormalities in basement membrane of inner ear, kidney, and retina
- *Branchio-oto-renal syndrome*—renal dysplasia/agenesis with abnormalities of branchial arches 1 and 2 causing. Variable hearing loss SNHL/conductive/mixed, malformed pinna/pre-auricular pits, branchial cleft cyst/fistula, lacrimal duct abnormalities.

4.5 How can we test a child's hearing and at what age can these tests be performed?

- *Objective tests*—tympanometry, OAE-evoked response audiometry
- *Subjective tests*—distraction test (6–24 months), visual response audiometry (6–24 months), play audiometry(>24 months), speech audiometry (2–5 years), pure tone audiometry (>5 years).

4.6 What investigations would you perform on an otherwise normal baby with audiologically-confirmed profound bilateral hearing loss? Please briefly state the rationale for each investigation.

- *Imaging*—MRI of inner ear/IAM and will show abnormalities of cranial nerve VII and VIII as well as membranous labyrinth and brain
- CT provides better bony detail including ossicles, but involves radiation
- It may be best to perform these early (<3 months) before sedation or even a general anaesthetic is required
- *Renal ultrasound*—indicated if branchio-oto-renal syndrome is suspected (i.e. pre-auricular pits, branchial sinuses)

- *Electrocardiogram (ECG)*—to detect for long QT as seen in Jervell Lange–Nielson syndrome. Although very rare, this is a simple non-invasive test to perform
- *Urinalysis*—blood and protein, as seen in Alport syndrome
- *Thyroid function tests (TFTs)*—(although likely to have been done postnatally) to exclude hypothyroidism as seen in Pendred's, U&Es (Alports), FBC rarely indicated
- *Ophthalmology review*—by paediatric ophthalmologist as 40% of children with permanent congenital hearing impairment have ophthalmic conditions and this may help make the diagnosis of a syndrome such as Usher or CHARGE
- *Congenital infection*—urine/saliva cytomegalovirus (CMV) DNA polymerase chain reaction (PCR; commonest intrauterine infection causing hearing loss in UK). If done early may allow treatment to prevent hearing loss with valgancyclovir
- *Rubella*—IgM in blood present for at least 3 months
- *Toxoplasma*—IgM present for 6 months
- Syphilis serology
- *Genetic testing:*
  - ◆ Connexin 26 and 30 mutations
  - ◆ *Pendrin* gene in enlarged vestibular aqueduct/Mondini
  - ◆ Chromosome abnormalities where there is suspected developmental delay or dysmorphic features
- Consider test for m.1555A>G mitochondrial mutation especially if hearing loss following aminoglycosides.

4.7 What is the benefit of investigating for an aetiology?

- To help parents understand cause of their child's deafness
- To provide better advice to parents for future family planning
- To identify and treat any infection early to prevent further hearing loss
- To identify and treat potentially serious associated complications, e.g. conduction defect and cardiac arrest in Jervell Lange–Nielson
- To provide better advice to parents, which may prevent further loss, such as avoiding exposure to aminoglycosides in m.1555A>G mutation or avoiding head trauma in enlarged vestibular aqueduct
- To determine best management options for rare conditions, such as aplastic auditory nerves.

Question 5

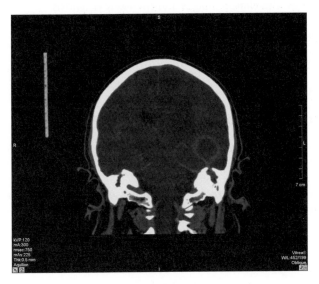

Figure 3.5.1

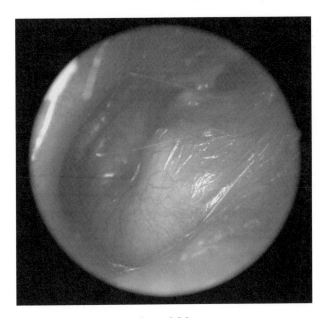

Figure 3.5.2

A 25-year-old female presents to A&E with a 6-day history of left otalgia and deafness, 3 days of headache and 24h of confusion. The images shown (Figures 3.5.1 and 3.5.2 (otoscopic image)) are from her initial examination and investigations.

5.1 Please describe the clinical images and the likely diagnosis.

5.2 How would you manage this patient?

5.3 How can you assess for meningism?

5.4 What are the most likely pathogens?

5.5 What are the complications of acute otitis media?

5.6 What are the potential routes of spread of intracranial infection from acute otitis media?

5.7 Where do Bezold's, Luc's, and Citelli's abscesses present, and what is the anatomical basis for their location?

Answers to Question 5

5.1 Please describe the clinical images and the likely diagnosis.

Coronal CT (with contrast) showing a ring enhancing intracranial lesion of low attenuation in the left temporal lobe with a corresponding defect in the tegmen of the temporal bone. The otoscopic image shows a bulging left tympanic membrane. The diagnosis is otogenic intracerebral abscess from acute otitis media.

5.2 How would you manage this patient?

The focus of care for this patient is treatment of the life threatening intracranial infection. Following an ABCD approach (to include Glasgow Coma Score (GCS)) and appropriate resuscitation, a focused history should include any previous otological disease/surgery. The examination should include a full neurological assessment. Broad spectrum intravenous antibiotics should be given early. This patient should be managed jointly with a neurosurgical team +/− intensive care unit (ITU; depending on GCS). This will require urgent transfer to a neurosurgical centre.

It is likely that with an abscess of this size, surgery will be required. This may require a combined neurosurgical/ENT procedure. Minimum surgery to the ear would comprise of myringotomy and grommet insertion. Often a cortical mastoidectomy and washout of middle ear will be performed with drain insertion. Pus should be sent at the time of surgery for microbial assessment. Formal exploration of the middle ear, if required, is usually delayed until the patient is stable.

5.3 How can you assess for meningism?

The classical triad for meningism is nuchal rigidity (neck stiffness) headache and photophobia. Specific tests include Kernig's and Brudzinski's signs.

5.4 What are the most likely pathogens?

The most common pathogens in acute otitis media are *Streptococcus pneumoniae*, *Haemophilus influenzae* and *Moraxella catarrhalis*. (Intracranial spread is often from *Streptococcus milleri*.)

5.5 What are the complications of acute otitis media?

Extracranial

- *Intratemporal:*
    - Tympanic membrane perforation
    - Acute mastoiditis
    - Tympanosclerosis
    - Hearing loss; conductive/sensorineural
    - chronic supporative otitis media (CSOM)/otitis media with effusion (OME)
    - Labyrinthitis
    - Facial nerve palsy
    - Petrositis
- *Extratemporal:*
    - Bezold's/Citelli's/Luc's abscess
    - Subperiosteal (mastoid) abscess.

Intracranial

- Meningitis

- Extradural abscess
- Subdural abscess
- Intracerebral abscess
- Sigmoid sinus thrombosis
- Otitic hydrocephalus.

Systemic

Embolic spread

5.6 What are the potential routes of spread of intracranial infection from acute otitis media?

- Direct spread from osteitis and bone erosion
- Lymphatic/haematogenous, i.e. venous channels
- Normal anatomical structures: oval/round window, cochlea, and vestibular aqueducts
- Spread through fracture lines or iatrogenic bony defects.

5.7 Where do Bezold's, Luc's, and Citelli's abscesses present and what is the anatomical basis for their location?

- A Bezold's abscess is a neck abscess associated with the sternocleidomastoid (SCM) muscle due to extension of mastoiditis through the mastoid tip along the SCM muscle (may be more posterior in neck)
- A Luc's abscess occurs at the root of the pneumatized zygoma
- A Citteli's abscess occurs when the mastoiditis extends through the mastoid tip, but tracks down the digastric muscle (may be more anterior in neck).

Question 6

A normally fit and well 70-year-old lady presents to the OPD with dizziness. Six weeks ago she developed sudden onset acute rotatory vertigo following an upper respiratory tract infection. There was associated nausea, but no hearing loss or tinnitus. This was continuous and severe for 2 days, during which time she was unable to walk. She still feels unsteady when walking especially at night or on uneven surfaces. In addition over the last few weeks she has developed brief (seconds) episodes of dizziness when turning over in bed.

6.1 When assessing this patient in clinic, what would you look for on examination?

6.2 Would you routinely perform any investigations?

6.3 What do you think caused her initial vertigo?

6.4 Why is she unsteady at night?

6.5 What is causing her dizziness turning over in bed and is this related to her initial episode of vertigo?

6.6 What is shown in Figure 3.6.1 and what are they for?

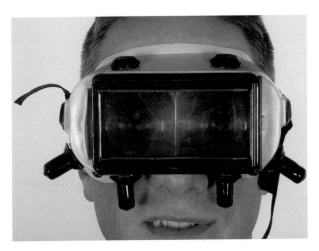

Figure 3.6.1

6.7 How can you test for severe unilateral vestibular hypofunction on examination?

6.8 What in the history would make you suspect bilateral vestibular failure and how would you test for it on examination?

6.9   How would you manage this patient?

6.10 What are the surgical options for treating a patient with posterior canal benign paroxysmal positional vertigo refractory to conservative measures?

Answers to Question 6

6.1 When assessing this patient in clinic, what would you look for on examination?

The neuro-otological examination is likely to include: otoscopy, tuning fork tests, cranial nerve exam, eye movements (saccades and smooth pursuit), head thrust, Romberg's/Unterberger's and Dix–Hallpike tests.

6.2 Would you routinely perform any investigations?

Routine

Pure tone audiogram (PTA): Some may consider vestibular function testing with calorics.

6.3 What do you think caused her initial vertigo?

Acute vestibular failure

Labyrinthitis/vestibular neuronitis/acute peripheral vestibulopathy.

6.4 Why is she unsteady at night?

Patients with vestibular hypofunction are more reliant on their visual and proprioceptive input to maintain their balance. Low light or uneven surfaces reduces this input and can result in imbalance.

6.5 What is causing her dizziness turning over in bed and is this related to her initial episode of vertigo?

These symptoms are typical for benign paroxysmal positional vertigo (BPPV). BPPV is known to occur in association with other labyrinthine disease/insult, such as head injury, vestibular neuronitis, or Ménière's disease.

6.6 What is shown in Figure 3.6.1 and what are they for?

Frenzel's goggles have magnifying glasses for lenses and have an internal light to illuminate the patient's eyes. This allows the eyes to be seen very clearly, making small movements easier to identify. The high magnification prevents the patient from focusing, thereby removing visual fixation and accentuating any previously undetected nystagmus.

6.7 How can you test for severe unilateral vestibular hypofunction on examination?

- Spontaneous nystagmus may rarely be present, especially if visual fixation is reduced by removal of glasses or wearing Frenzel glasses
- The 'head-thrust test' tests the vestibulo-ocular reflex
- Unterberger test may identify rotation towards the side of vestibular hypofunction.

6.8 What in the history would make you suspect bilateral vestibular failure and how would you test for it on examination?

Bobbing oscillopsia or visual blurring on walking/running/driving is suggestive. Head-thrust test will be abnormal in both directions. Dynamic visual acuity involves testing visual acuity with a LogMar or Snellen chart (using both eyes) then repeating this, whilst oscillating the head from side to side. Reduced visual acuity by more than 3 lines on the chart is highly suggestive of loss of vestibulo-ocular reflex function. LogMar chart is displayed in Figure 3.6.2.

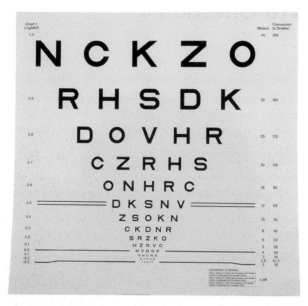

Figure 3.6.2 LogMar chart.

6.9 How would you manage this patient?

Her BPPV can be treated with an Epley or Semont manoeuvre. Her unilateral vestibulopathy can be treated with vestibular rehabilitation.

6.10 What are the surgical options for treating a patient with posterior canal benign paroxysmal positional vertigo refractory to conservative measures?

Posterior canal occlusion/obliteration. Singular nerve section is no longer indicated due to high risk of SNHL.

Question 7

Figure 3.7.1 shows an MRI head of a 24-year-old female.

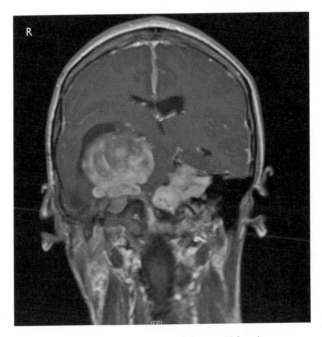

Figure 3.7.1 MRI head of a 24-year-old female

7.1 Please describe the abnormalities shown in this scan.

7.2 What is the likely underlying diagnosis?

7.3 What are the other hallmark features of this and what is the usual age of onset?

7.4 What is the pathogenesis of this condition?

7.5 What is the inheritability of this condition?

7.6 Is genetic counseling helpful in this condition?

7.7 How should a new diagnosis be evaluated?

7.8 In a patient who has previously undergone surgical removal of a right-sided vestibular schwannoma, leaving them with a profound hearing loss on that side, how would you manage their hearing rehabilitation if the contralateral side was due to undergo excision of an acoustic neuroma?

Answers to Question 7

7.1 Please describe the abnormalities shown in this scan.

T1 MRI (probably post-gadolinium contrast) showing bilateral enhancing masses in CPA with extension into IAM (more so on the right) and displacement of brainstem to the right. Likely bilateral vestibular schwannomas.

7.2 What is the likely underlying diagnosis?

Neurofibromatosis Type 2.

7.3 What are the other hallmark features of this and what is the usual age of onset?

Bilateral vestibular schwannomas (diagnostic for NF2), other cranial nerve schwannomas and meningiomas, posterior subcapsular lenticular opacities (cataracts), spinal tumours, skin tumours/lesions.

The average age of onset of the condition is 18–24 years with most developing bilateral vestibular schwanomma (VS) by the age of 30 years. Rarely, it may present after 60 years of age.

7.4 What is the pathogenesis of this condition?

NF2 arises due to a mutation in the *Merlin* gene on chromosome 22. The Merlin protein belongs to a family of proteins that are involved in regulating cell–cell interactions. It is thought that loss of this protein may lead to loss of contact inhibition and, therefore, resultant tumorogenesis.

The *NF2* gene defect has been identified in other neoplastic conditions, such as meningiomas and colorectal tumours.

7.5 What is the inheritability of this condition?

NF2 has an autosomal dominant pattern of inheritance with >95% penetrance, although in 50% of cases there is no family history and this represents a new mutation.

7.6 Is genetic counseling helpful in this condition?

Yes

- Genetic testing is possible for those relatives at risk
- This allows for surveillance of at-risk individuals with annual MRI scanning from aged 10 years until mid-adult life
- In addition, it may be possible to offer prenatal testing of at risk pregnancies if the specific mutation is known. This is done with chorionic villous sampling or amniocentesis.

7.7 How should a new diagnosis be evaluated?

NF2 should ideally be evaluated and managed in a designated NF2 specialist centre. New cases should undergo, at least, head MRI, audiological assessment, including auditory brainstem response (ABR), ophthalmological assessment, cutaneous examination, genetics consultation.

7.8 In a patient who has previously undergone surgical removal of a right-sided vestibular schwannoma, leaving them with a profound hearing loss on that side, how would you manage their hearing rehabilitation if the contralateral side was due to undergo excision of an acoustic neuroma?

Surgery should be avoided if at all possible in the only hearing ear. Gamma knife radiotherapy to stabilize the tumour may be appropriate. If surgery is necessary, this may be combined with insertion of an auditory brainstem implant.

Question 8

8.1 Describe the CT shown in Figure 3.8.1.

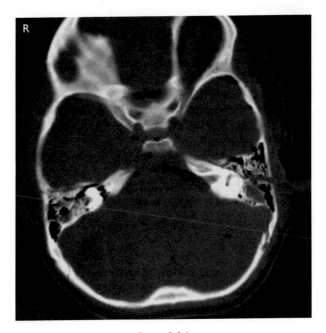

Figure 3.8.1

8.2 Describe your initial management of this patient.

8.3 Give a classification of such injuries, their mechanism of injury, and their sequelae.

8.4 Describe the CT shown in Figure 3.8.2. Using the previous classification, what
type of injury is this likely to represent?

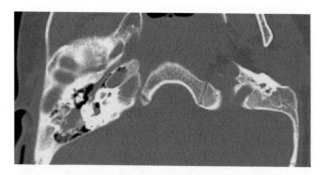

Figure 3.8.2

Answers to Question 8

8.1 Describe the CT shown in Figure 3.8.1.

There is a longitudinal fracture line, which extends to involve both temporal bones (more anterior on the right) probably affecting the roof of the external auditory meatus to the tympanic membrane and the roof of the middle ear. There is marked pneumocephalus throughout the cranium.

8.2 Describe your initial management of this patient.

The initial management of patients with a temporal bone fracture should include identification and treatment of any associated serious or life-threatening injuries. Temporal bone fractures usually result from a significant force of impact and, therefore, the possibility of an associated intracranial haemorrhage or c-spine injury is high. With this in mind:

- ABC (to include GCS)/resuscitation
- General head injury and c-spine management by appropriate teams
- Specific examination of the ears, facial nerve and tuning fork tests +/− PTA
- The role of prophylactic antibiotics to reduce subsequent intracranial infection, is controversial
- Ear injuries are usually managed conservatively in the first instance
- The main exception to this is a clear history of immediate total facial nerve lower motor neurone palsy (LMN) injury, depending on CT findings-consider exploration of the nerve by otoneurosurgeon.

8.3 Give a classification of such injuries, their mechanism of injury, and their sequelae.

Temporal bone fractures are traditionally classified into longitudinal or transverse, depending on orientation of fracture line to the long axis of the petrous temporal bone. In actual fact most are a mixture of the two, but may be predominantly longitudinal or transverse. Alternatively, they can be classified as either involving or sparing the otic capsule. This may be more helpful in predicting the likely sequelae, but is less commonly used in practice.

Longitudinal fractures

80%, usually due to blow to side of head. Fracture usually runs from the squamous portion medially along roof of external auditory canal, middle ear cleft, and on into the petrous apex, potentially to involve the foramen lacerum or foramen ovale. Symptoms mainly related to middle ear as the otic capsule is rarely involved. This may result in:

- Laceration in external auditory canal (EAC) skin or rupture of tympanic membrane causing bleeding from ear
- Conductive hearing loss from blood in EAC, haemotympanum, or disruption of the ossicular chain
- Sensorineural hearing loss may occur, but is typically not severe and may be temporary due to cochlear concussion
- CSF otorrhoea or otorhinorroea if canal and TM intact
- Facial nerve injury rare (usually neuropraxia or axonotmesis).

Transverse fractures

20%, usually from blow to front or back of skull.

Fracture runs **across** long axis of petrous bone and is much more likely to involve otic capsule and IAM. Symptoms mainly related to inner ear injury.

- Haemotympanum as TM often intact
- Facial nerve injury (LMN), occurs in 50% of transverse fractures and often immediate
- Otic capsule disruption (irreversible SNHL, dead ear, severe vertigo).

8.4 Describe the CT shown in Figure 3.8.2. Using the previous classification, what type of injury is this likely to represent?

Opacification within the right mastoid, but most importantly pneumolabyrinth (as well as air adjacent to the internal carotid artery (ICA) in foramen lacerum/carotid canal). Pneumolabyrinth is indicative of otic capsule disruption and is often accompanied by SNHL and severe vertigo (most common with transverse fracture). Management is conservative in most cases.

Question 9

Figure 3.9.1 shows a red/blue mass behind the TM.

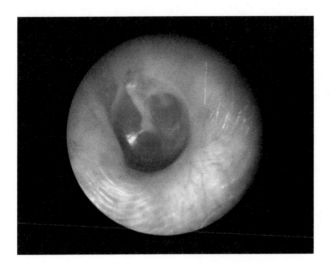

Figure 3.9.1

9.1 Give the possible causes for a red/blue mass behind the TM?

9.2 How might this patient present?

9.3 From what tissue do these tumours arise?

9.4 Where else can these tumours arise in the head and neck?

9.5 How would you investigate this patient?

9.6 Do you know any way of classifying these lesions?

9.7 If limited to the mesotympanum how would you manage this patient?

9.8 Where is the blood supply to these tumours usually from?

9.9 If arising from the jugular foramen how would you manage this patient and what are the principal steps in surgery to this location?

9.10 From where does one encounter problematic bleeding during excision of a lesion affecting the jugular foramen?

Answers to Question 9

9.1 Give the possible causes for a red/blue mass behind the TM.

Otoendoscopic image of a left ear with a red/purple mass behind the mesotympanic TM. Likely representing a paraganglioma; glomus tympanicum (or possibly glomus jugulare, although appears centred on promontory). Other possible causes for a red/blue mass behind the TM include aberrant ICA, high riding/dehiscent jugular bulb, other middle ear neoplasm (haemangioma, adenoma, malignancy), persistent stapedial artery, Schwarzte sign, granuloma, etc.

9.2 How might this patient present?

Most commonly pulsatile tinnitus and conductive hearing loss if confined to the mesotympanum. Skull base involvement, especially glomus jugulare tumours may cause lower cranial nerve palsies, such as IX, X, XI, and XII. (SNHL, vertigo and palsies of CN VII and VI are less common, but possible depending on direction of growth).

9.3 From what tissue do these tumours arise?

Paragangliomas arise from chemoreceptor (or paraganglionic) tissue associated with the autonomic nervous system. Embryologically, this tissue is derived from neural crest cells.

9.4 Where else can these tumours arise in the head and neck?

The commonest site for a paraganglioma is a carotid body tumour, but paragangliomas of the vagus nerve may also occur.

9.5 How would you investigate this patient?

PTA/tympanometry. CT temporal bone to assess bony erosion. MRI to assess for intracranial extension with typical 'salt and pepper' appearance due to flow voids from high vascularity. Twenty-four hours urinary catecholamine collection to exclude the 1–3% chance of this being a secreting tumour or an associated phaeochromocytoma. Angiography can be helpful diagnostically to confirm the vascular nature of the lesion, assess for collateral circulation (carotid balloon occlusion test), as well as to guide pre-operative embolization.

Box 3.9.1 **Fisch classification**

- Type A tumour limited to middle ear
- Type B tumour in middle ear and mastoid with no destruction of bone of infralabyrinthine compartment
- Type C tumour invading bone of infralabyrinthine compartment and extending to petrous apex
- Type D tumour with intracranial extension.

Reproduced from Fisch U. The infratemporal fossa approach for nasopharyngeal tumors. *Laryngoscope* **93**: 36–44. Copyright 1983, with permission of John Wiley and Sons.

9.6 Do you know any way of classifying these lesions?

The Fisch classification of middle ear glomus tumours is as shown in Box 3.9.1.

There is also the Glasscock–Jackson classification, which differentiates between tympanicum and jugulare tumours.

9.7 If limited to the mesotympanum how would you manage this patient?

Small glomus tympanicum tumours can be simply excised via a standard tympanotomy (percanal/post-auricular/endaural), often with the aid of a laser or diathermy.

9.8 Where is the blood supply to these tumours usually from?

Ascending pharyngeal artery.

9.9 If arising from the jugular foramen how would you manage this patient and what are the principal steps in surgery to this location?

The management of glomus jugulare tumours depends on tumour factors and patient factors/comorbidities. Options include monitoring with serial scans, radiation therapy (to arrest growth), embolization, and surgical excision. In these tumours, surgery carries a significant risk of facial palsy, aspiration, and dysphagia, meaning radiotherapy may be preferred as an initial treatment option.

Surgery is usually preceded by embolization and is performed via a transtemporal skull base or infratemporal fossa approach. Surgical steps usually include:

- Dissection of the neck and control of internal jugular vein (IJV) and carotid (ICA/external carotid artery (ECA))
- Identification of CN VII in parotid gland
- Extended cortical mastoidectomy
- Control of sigmoid sinus and ligation of IJV
- Dissection of tumour
- Blind sac closure.

9.10 From where does one encounter problematic bleeding during excision of a lesion affecting the jugular foramen?

Bleeding can occur from several sites, but is usually controllable. Removal of the tumour from the jugular foramen can be associated with brisk bleeding from the inferior petrosal sinus, which may only be stopped with packing once the tumour is removed.

Question 10

10.1 How common is congenital deafness?

10.2 How is this usually identified and what are the advantages of early detection?

10.3 When and where is hearing screening carried out?

10.4 What risk factors for congenital deafness would be important in the history of a neonate?

10.5 Which tests are used for screening?

10.6 What is auditory neuropathy?

Answers to Question 10

10.1 How common is congenital deafness?

1–2 per 1000 well babies. (10–20 times higher in the neonatal intensive care unit (NICU)/special care baby unit (SCBU) population, i.e. 1 in 100).

10.2 How is this usually identified and what are the advantages of early detection?

In the UK, the Newborn Hearing Screening Programme (NHSP) tests all newborns, and aims to diagnose and treat hearing loss early, as this leads to improved speech, language, and social development for children.

10.3 When and where is hearing screening carried out?

This may be carried out either in the hospital setting postnatally prior to discharge or in the community at the primary health visitor birth visit age 10 days. Ideally, screening should be completed by 4–5 weeks of age, but may be done up to 3 months of age.

Screening should be carried out by 'screeners' specifically employed to carry out hearing screening who are usually a paediatric nurse or health visitor.

N.B. Do not test before 34 weeks gestational age as the auditory system may still be immature.

10.4 What risk factors for congenital deafness would be important in the history of a neonate?

- Family history of congenital hearing loss, consanguinity
- Maternal illness/poor health e.g. DM/alcohol excess
- Proven or possible perinatal infection with TORCH e.g. Cytomegalovirus, Rubella or toxoplasmosis
- Birth difficulties e.g. APGAR scores suggesting hypoxia/asphyxia
- Neonatal intensive care unit (NICU)/special care baby unit (SCBU) for >48 h especially if IPPV
- Neonatal jaundice/hyperbilirubinaemia
- Meningitis (1 in 10 develop SNHL)
- Ototoxic medication (especially outside therapeutic levels)
- Craniofacial abnormalities including Down's syndrome.

10.5 Which tests are used for screening?

For 'well babies', an automated oto-acoustic emission (AOAE) is performed in the first instance and if abnormal after a second attempt (at a second sitting), an automated auditory brainstem response (AABR) is tested. If one or both ears fail to give a clear response, the child is referred early for audiological assessment at a specialist centre.

For babies who have spent >48 hours in NICU/SCBU there is a separate protocol for screening that involves performing both AOAE and ABR on all babies. The rationale for this is that these babies have a higher chance of auditory neuropathy or dys-synchrony, which might be missed if only an AOAE is performed.

Babies with risk factors for hearing loss will also be tested using the NICU/SCBU protocol.

10.6 What is auditory neuropathy?

Auditory neuropathy is a disorder that affects the neural processing of auditory stimuli.

It is thought to occur in up to 1 in 10 children who have a hearing loss and a severely abnormal ABR, although the true prevalence is unknown. The cause is also unknown, but it is more common in children who had neonatal problems, such as prematurity, hypoxia, or jaundice.

The hallmark is of very abnormal or absent ABR with normal OAEs. The management is careful observation and assessment, hearing aids, and early behavioural testing to establish behavioral thresholds. Speech/language development must be monitored and if delayed, the child should be considered for cochlear implantation.

Question 11

A 4-year-old boy is referred by his GP with parental concerns regarding his hearing. Otoscopy has a similar appearance bilaterally and shows a yellowish hue to the drum, with fluid bubbles evident. Tympanometry shows a flat trace (Type B) and audiometry is shown in Figure 3.11.1.

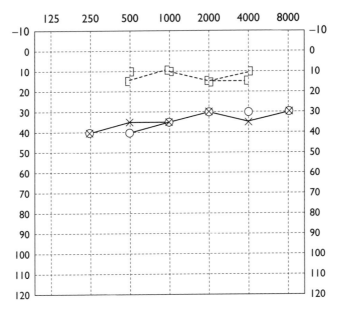

Figure 3.11.1

11.1 What is the likely diagnosis?

11.2 What are the risk factors for this condition?

11.3 What are the other important points in the history?

11.4 What would be your initial management for this patient?

11.5 If the symptoms are persistent, what are the management options?

11.6 What are the indications for grommet insertion?

11.7 How does your management of this condition change in patients with Down's syndrome and why? What about in patients with cleft palate?

11.8 What is the role of adenoidectomy in the management of this condition?

11.9 How do grommets work?

Answers to Question 11

11.1 What is the likely diagnosis?

Otitis media with effusion (OME)/glue ear.

11.2 What are the risk factors for this condition?

Patient factors

- Age <5, atopy (e.g. allergic rhinitis), reflux, family history
- Anatomical; craniofacial abnormalities (including Down's syndrome and cleft palate)
- Physiological; Kartagener/cystic fibrosis.

Enviromental factors

Parental smoking, absence of breastfeeding, early day care nursery, multiple siblings.

11.3 What are the other important points in the history?

Duration of symptoms, ear infections, speech and language development, behavioural difficulties, co-existing medical conditions.

11.4 What would be your initial management for this patient?

Watchful waiting is the first line of management for patients with a new diagnosis of otitis media with effusion (OME) as 50% of children will have resolution in symptoms by 3 months.

11.5 If the symptoms are persistent, what are the management options?

- Further watchful waiting as 95% resolve after 1 year
- *Auto-inflation techniques/devices*—otovent balloon (£7.00). Good evidence to show short-term benefit in some patients, but long-term effects not known (van den Aardweg et al., 2010)
- *Ventilation tubes/grommets*—these remain the most effective treatment option for persistent OME with hearing loss. Most of the improvement in hearing compared with controls is seen in the 6–9 months following insertion
- *Hearing aids*—these are a viable alternative to managing the hearing loss in OME; however, they are not always well tolerated. In addition, hearing loss can fluctuate in OME, and hearing aids may need frequent adjustments
- There is no evidence to support the use of other medical therapies in the treatment of OME.

11.6 What are the indications for grommet insertion?

- Bilateral OME documented over a period of 3 months with a hearing level in the better ear of 25–30dBHL or worse averaged at 0.5, 1, 2, and 4kHz
- Recurrent acute otitis media (AOM)
- Acutely when treating complications of AOM, e.g. facial palsy, mastoiditis.

11.7 How does your management of this condition change in patients with Down's syndrome and why? What about in patients with cleft palate?

In general, most patients with Down's syndrome should be offered hearing aids as first line instead of grommets (NICE, 2008). The rationale for this is that they are more likely to develop otorrhoea, extrude grommets early, insertion may be technically difficult or impossible due to narrow canals, and they may have additional co-existing permanent conductive or SNHL requiring hearing aids even after grommet insertion.

Cleft palate

Again, NICE guidance from 2008 suggests that although each patient should have an individual assessment, many will be managed with hearing aids. As with Down's syndrome, patients with a cleft palate are at increased risk of persistent/recurrent OME and if treated with grommets may require multiple insertions throughout their childhood.

11.8 What is the role of adenoidectomy in the management of this condition?

A Cochrane review from 2009 (van den Aardweg et al., 2010) showed a significant benefit of adenoidectomy regarding the resolution of OME in children. However, the benefit to hearing is small and the effects on changes in the tympanic membrane are unknown. The risks of operating should be weighed against these potential benefits. The absence of a significant benefit of adenoidectomy on AOM suggests that routine surgery for this indication is not warranted.

NICE (2008) recommends that adjuvant adenoidectomy should not be used in the absence of recurrent/persistent upper respiratory tract symptoms.

Most clinicians would reserve adjuvant adenoidectomy for patients requiring a second set of grommets or those with an independent indication, such as nasal block from adenoidal hypertrophy.

11.9 How do grommets work?

Grommets ventilate the middle ear. They reduce middle ear hypoxia, and allow clearance of effusion. The mechanism of action is unknown. Grommets do not resolve the underlying cause of the OME.

Further reading

NICE Guideline CG60 (2008). *Surgical management of children with otitis media with effusion (OME)*. London: National Institute for Health and Clinical Excellence. Available at: http://guidance.nice.org.uk/CG60.

van den Aardweg MTA, Schilder AGM, Herkert E, Boonacker CWB, Rovers MM (2010). Adenoidectomy for otitis media in children. *Cochrane Database of System Rev* Issue 1, Art. No.: CD007810.

Question 12

A 43-year-old woman presents to clinic with a 1-year history of episodic vertigo lasting 2–3 hours associated with tinnitus, hearing loss, and a preceding sensation of aural fullness on the right. Weber (512Hz) test lateralizes to the left, with Rinne test positive bilaterally. Her audiogram is shown in Figure 3.12.1.

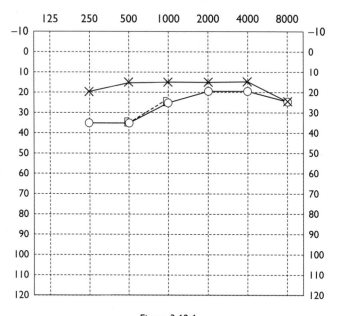

Figure 3.12.1

12.1 What is the likely diagnosis?

12.2 Which investigations may help to clarify the diagnosis?

12.3 Do you know any way of classifying the certainty of your diagnosis?

12.4 What are the management options for patients with this condition?

12.5 What should you advise this lady regarding driving her car?

12.6 What is a crisis of Tumarkins?

12.7 How is electrocochleography performed, what does it measure and what are its potential uses?

Answers to Question 12

12.1 What is the likely diagnosis?

Ménière's disease.

12.2 Which investigations may help to clarify the diagnosis?

The diagnosis of Ménière's disease is usually made on clinical grounds, including at least one PTA. However, often additional investigations are considered to rule out other differential diagnoses, which may have a similar presentation.

- *Imaging*—MRI to exclude acoustic neuroma
- *Blood tests*—consider autoimmune profile and syphilis serology
- Other investigations may also be considered especially in the research setting:
  - *Electrocochleography (ECoG)*—to detect an increase in the ratio of summating potential to action potential (SP/AP >0.5)
  - *Calorics*—may detect a canal paresis in the affected ear
  - *Glycerol dehydration test*—oral glycerol is ingested (or mannitol), which acts as an osmotic diuretic. In the presence of cochlear hydrops, this can lead to an improvement in their PTA/speech audiometry/ECoG. (Sensitivity ~50% and rarely done because of risk of complications.)

12.3 Do you know any way of classifying the certainty of your diagnosis?

AAO-HNS Committee on Hearing and Equilibrium revised definition in 1995:

- *Possible Ménière's disease*—typical episodic vertigo without documented hearing loss *or* SNHL (fluctuating or fixed) with disequilibrium, but no definitive episodes of vertigo
- *Probable Ménière's disease*—one definitive episode of vertigo + audiometrically-documented hearing loss on at least one occasion + tinnitus or aural fullness in the affected ear
- *Definite Ménière's disease*—two or more definitive spontaneous episodes of vertigo for 20min or longer, + audiometrically-documented hearing loss on at least one occasion, + tinnitus or aural fullness in the affected ear
- *Certain Ménière's disease*—definite Ménière's disease, plus histopathological confirmation.

12.4 What are the management options for patients with this condition?

There is a lack of good evidence for most treatments in Ménière's, but in general they include:

Conservative

- *Patient education and counselling*—leaflet, Ménière's society website, reassurance, stress management/relaxation
- *Life style measures*—reduction of dietary salt, fluid, caffeine, alcohol, and smoking
- Hearing aid for hearing loss
- Tinnitus management.

Medical

- Betahistine aims to improve middle ear blood flow and is used to reduce the frequency of attacks (benefit shown in several trials, but not high quality)
- Vestibular sedatives such as prochlorperazine can be used to control acute attacks of vertigo

- Diuretics (Burgess & Kundu, 2006 showed no good evidence to support this)
- Intratympanic steroids (benefit shown in single study reported in Phillips & Westerberg, July 2011).

Surgical—hearing preservation

- Grommet insertion +/− Meniett device
- Endolymphatic sac decompression (controversial)
- Vestibular nerve section (requires craniotomy).

Surgical—non-hearing preservation *(most effective)*

- Intratympanic gentamicin ablation therapy may be regarded as potentially preserving hearing, but with repeated doses the risk of hearing loss increases and may be as high as 15–30%
- Labyrinthectomy is very effective at resolving vertiginous attacks, but causes complete hearing loss and vestibular failure, which may cause disabling permanent dysequilibrium if there is contralateral vestibular hypofunction.

12.5 What should you advise this lady regarding driving her car?

The Driver and Vehicle Licensing Authority (DVLA) guidelines (revised in May 2012) state that patients 'liable to sudden attacks of unprovoked or unprecipitated disabling giddiness' should cease driving and contact the DVLA on diagnosis. However, this patient, like many patients with Ménière's disease, has a preceding warning symptom of aural fullness prior to the onset of vertigo and does not therefore fall into the above DVLA patient group. Therefore, providing she has sufficient warning of her attacks she should be safe to continue driving.

12.6 What is a crisis of Tumarkins?

This is a type of 'drop attack' affecting ~2% of patients with Ménière's disease caused by sudden loss of extensor function without loss of consciousness and with complete recovery. It is likely to relate to involvement of the otolith organs and will have implications regarding driving safety (usually drop attacks do not occur while seated, in which case driving is possible).

12.7 How is electrocochleography performed, what does it measure and what are its potential uses?

ECochG is an objective test, which measures the electrical output of the cochlea and auditory nerve in response to an auditory stimulus. One major advantage of the test is that it does not require masking.

The patient lies in a soundproof room with a ground electrode on the forehead and a reference electrode on the ipsilateral mastoid process. The active electrode is ideally placed in contact with the promontory (transtympanic), but ear canal electrodes may also be used. A sound stimulus (such as wide band click) is presented to the ear and the electrical response is measured for 10ms. The resultant compound action potential consists of:

- Cochlear microphonic (CM), originating from the basilar membrane indicating the hair cells are intact
- SP, also originating from the hair cells, is an alteration in the electrical potential baseline. This is used in the diagnosis of Ménière's
- AP, electrical response of the auditory nerve used for determining thresholds (similar to wave I in ABR)

- ECochG may be useful for:
  - Diagnosis of Ménière's (SP/AP >0.5)
  - Accurate objective measure of threshold determination but only for frequencies 3–4kH. Therefore, useful when conventional subjective audiometry is inadequate, such as in non-organic hearing loss or bilateral severe mixed hearing loss where bone conduction thresholds cannot be adequately masked
  - Intra-operative monitoring during surgery around IAM/inner ear.

Further reading

Burgess A, Kundu S (2006). Diuretics for Ménière's disease or syndrome. *Cochrane Database System Rev*, Issue 3. Art. No.: CD003599.

DVLA (2012). *At a Glance Guide to the Current Medical Standards of Fitness to Drive*, revised May 2012. Swansea: DVLA. Available at: http://www.dft.gov.uk/dvla/medical/aag.aspx

Committee on Hearing and Equilibrium (1995). Guidelines for the diagnosis and evaluation of therapy in Meniere's disease. *Am Acad Otolaryngol-Head Neck Found, Otolaryngol-Head Neck Surg* **113**(3)**:** 181–5.

Phillips JS, Westerberg B (2011). Intratympanic steroids for Ménière's disease or syndrome. *Cochrane Database System Rev*, Issue 7. Art. No.: CD008514.

Question 13

A 60-year-old man presents to clinic with gradually increasing hearing difficulties. Otoscopy is normal. His PTA is shown in Figure 3.13.1.

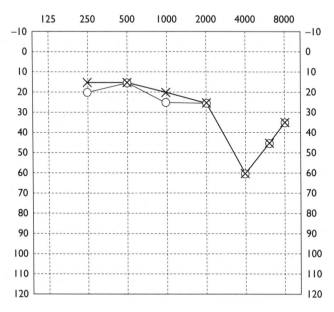

Figure 3.13.1 Patient's PTA.

13.1 Describe this audiogram.

13.2 What are the key points in the otological history to help identify the aetiology of hearing loss?

13.3 What is the most likely aetiology given this pattern of audiogram and what is the pathogenesis?

13.4 Why is the hearing loss worse at certain frequencies?

13.5 What is a temporary threshold shift?

13.6 Why are explosive or unexpected sounds potentially so damaging to the inner ear?

13.7 What legislation exists to protect employees working in a potentially noisy environment?

13.8 In a patient complaining of unilateral hearing loss due to occupational noise exposure, how would you investigate the possibility of non-organic hearing loss?

Answers to Question 13

13.1 Describe this audiogram.

Bilateral symmetrical high frequency hearing loss, which is worse at 4kHz.

13.2 What are the key points in the otological history to help identify the aetiology of hearing loss?

Other otological symptoms (tinnitus, vertigo), prior otological disease (i.e. infections, surgery), family history, medication (including chemotherapy), serious illnesses/infections, occupation, noise exposure.

13.3 What is the most likely aetiology given this pattern of audiogram and what is the pathogenesis?

This is likely to represent noise-induced hearing loss (NIHL). Prolonged and repeated exposure to loud noise (>85dB) causes mechanical and metabolic stress to most cell types within the inner ear, especially outer hair cells. This can lead to both temporary and permanent damage to inner ear cells.

13.4 Why is the hearing loss worse at certain frequencies?

Loud noise presented to the cochlea will affect the basal turn predominantly and therefore damage the highest frequencies. The natural resonant frequency of the middle ear and ossicles is 1–4kHz, meaning maximal energy transfer will be between these frequencies. It is likely that a combination of these two factors give rise to maximal loss and the 'notch' between 3 and 6kHz.

13.5 What is a temporary threshold shift?

This is noise-induced SNHL which resolves after 24–48h, although repeated temporary threshold shifts (TTS) may give rise to permanent threshold shift (PTS).

13.6 Why are explosive or unexpected sounds potentially so damaging to the inner ear?

The acoustic reflex provides some protection to the cochlea from continuous loud noise exposure as it is triggered by noises louder than 90dB. However, the reflex arc has a latency of 25–150ms meaning a sudden onset high intensity noise (explosion) may reach the cochlea before the acoustic reflex is activated causing immediate irreversible hearing loss.

13.7 What legislation exists to protect employees working in a potentially noisy environment?

The Control of Noise at Work Regulations 2005 Legislation sets out standards for employers (see Table 3.13.1).

Occupational NIHL became a compensable disorder in 1975. Claims can be made on an individual basis with assessment of disability supported by PTA findings.

13.8 In a patient complaining of unilateral hearing loss due to occupational noise exposure, how would you investigate the possibility of non-organic hearing loss?

One must have a high index of suspicion to diagnose non-organic hearing loss (NOHL). The index of suspicion may be raised in adults claiming for compensation or a child with emotional/psychological disturbance.

Initial clinical assessment may provide clues. Apparent hearing in clinic room better than PTA thresholds, patients complaining of a unilateral hearing loss may deny hearing the tuning fork placed on the ipsilateral mastoid when they would be expected to perceive the sound in the contralateral cochlea.

	Average SPL over 8 hours (A-weighted)	Peak SPL (C-weighted)	Action legally required by employer
Lower exposure limit	80dB	135dB	Assess risk to workers (monitor employee hearing levels and monitor work place noise levels) Provide information and training
Upper exposure limit	85dB	137dB	As above Provide hearing protection Provide 'Hearing Zones'
Exposure limit value	87dB	140dB	Employees should not be exposed

SPL, sound pressure level.

Data from *Noise at work: Guidance for employers on the Control of Noise at Work Regulations 2005*, INDG362(rev1). Published by the Health and Safety Executive, 2005.

Table 3.13.1 Control of Noise at Work Regulations 2005 Legislation

Subjective

- *Pure tone audiometry*—patients feigning hearing loss may give inconsistent results. The most common pattern of hearing loss that seems to be feigned is a flat audiogram with thresholds between 40 and 50dB. In addition, they may again claim not to hear unmasked bone conduction when, in fact, their contralateral cochlea thresholds are normal
- *Stenger's test*—tuning fork or audiometrically tested
- *Speech audiometry*—patients find it more difficult to exaggerate their impairment with speech audiometry than PTA
- *Delayed speech feedback*—the patient reads aloud and their speech is played back into the affected ear. If the patient can hear they are likely to hesitate or stutter.

Objective

- *Acoustic reflexes*—the stapedial reflex threshold is usually stimulated at 70–90dB above the pure tone threshold (although this is variable with recruitment). Certainly stapedial reflex thresholds within 20dB of apparent PTA thresholds make NOHL likely
- OAEs
- *Electrical response audiometry*—cortical electrical response audiometry (CERA) and ABR. CERA has the advantage that it is the most accurate for detecting different frequency thresholds, but requires a co-operative patient.

Further reading

The Health and Safety Executive (2005). *Noise at work: guidance for employers on the Control of Noise at Work Regulations 2005*, INDG362 (rev). London: Health and Safety Executive.

Question 14

A 27-year-old female presents to clinic with a unilateral right-sided 45dB conductive hearing loss and a history of occasional otorrhoea after swimming. The left ear is normal, the right shown in Figure 3.14.1.

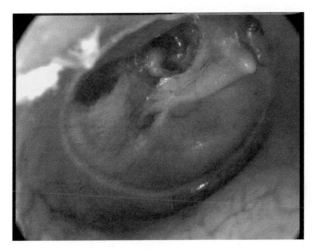

Figure 3.14.1

14.1 Please describe the image in Figure 3.14.1.

14.2 Is this a common ossicular abnormality? Why?

14.3 What are the management options for this patient?

14.4 In your pre-operative assessment, are there any non-audiological factors that would provide an indication as to the likely success of a tympanoplasty/ ossiculoplasty?

14.5 What is the definition of tympanoplasty? Do you know any ways of classifying tympanoplasty?

At subsequent outpatient review 1 year later, an obvious cholesteatoma was visible and the patient agrees to surgical treatment.

14.6 When planning surgery, what are the arguments for and against performing a preoperative CT scan?

Answers to Question 14

14.1 Please describe the image in Figure 3.14.1.

Posterosuperior pars tensa retraction pocket onto the head of stapes with absence of the long process of the incus. Anterior pars tensa well ventilated. Attic not clearly seen.

14.2 Is this a common ossicular abnormality? Why?

Yes. Propensity to erosion of the long/lenticular process of the incus is thought to be due to a poor blood supply.

14.3 What are the management options for this patient?

Conservative

- Education
- Water precautions to reduce otorrhoea
- Hearing aid to treat hearing loss.

Surgical

Tympanoplasty to resect retraction pocket and reconstruct (+/− reinforce with cartilage) to reduce risk of otorrhoea, prevent progression of disease and improve hearing.

14.4 In your pre-operative assessment, are there any non-audiological factors, which would provide an indication as to the likely success of a tympanoplasty/ossiculoplasty?

Middle ear ventilation is a key determining factor in success of ossiculoplasty. Therefore, if the ipsilateral anterior pars tensa is normal and the contralateral ear is well ventilated; this suggests good candidacy. Conversely, if the whole of the pars tensa is retracted and adherent in both ears, the chance of long-term success is reduced.

14.5 What is the definition of tympanoplasty? Do you know any ways of classifying tympanoplasty?

Tympanoplasty is an operation that aims to eradicate middle ear disease and reconstruct the hearing mechanism from the resulting defect. Classification as described by Wullstein (1953) (see Table 3.14.1).

14.6 When planning surgery, what are the arguments for and against performing a pre-operative CT scan?

Diagnosis of cholesteatoma is clinical, but CT scanning is helpful in planning treatment. Parameters that can be assessed include ossicular erosion, otic capsule fistula, facial canal dehiscence, tegmen dehiscence, mastoid size/pneumatization, presence of a dominant sigmoid sinus, and extent of disease.

Pros of CT scanning

This information may help guide a surgeon's choice of operation. If the CT shows a very small, poorly pneumatized mastoid with an anterior sigmoid sinus and low tegmen, the surgeon may choose to perform an attico-antrostomy or small cavity canal wall down procedure, when they might have normally performed a combined approach tympanoplasty (CAT). In addition, although CT cannot differentiate between different soft tissue densities in the middle ear and mastoid, if the mastoid is air filled, it may be possible to see that the disease is limited to the attic and tailor the surgery accordingly.

Type	Defect	Reconstruction
1	Isolated TM perforation	Reconstruct TM in presence of intact ossicular chain
2	Malleus handle absent	TM reconstructed over malleus remnant to lie on long process of incus
3	Absent malleus and incus	TM reconstructed with strut to head of stapes
4	Mobile stapes footplate (all other ossicles/stapes superstructure absent)	Recreate TM and separate oval window and round window by draping TM over superior promontory to create a round window baffle.
5	Fixed stapes footplate (all other ossicles/stapes superstructure absent)	Fenestration of the lateral semicircular canal is performed
6* (This type was added by Garcia Ibanez in 1961)	Ossicular discontinuity	Round window niche is left uncovered and TM reconstructed so that inferior edge lies on promontory above the round window creating oval window baffle

Reproduced from Wullstein H. Technic and early results of tympanoplasty. *Monatsschr Ohrenheilkd Laryngorhinol* **87**(4): 308–11.

Table 3.14.1 Wullstein classification

The sensitivity and specificity for CT identification of abnormalities, such as fistula or facial nerve dehiscence may be low. However, if a suspicion is raised on CT, it certainly increases the likelihood of the abnormality truly being present. Prior knowledge of this will allow particular care to be taken during certain points in the operation, but will also provide additional information on the risks of surgery.

With the increase in patient involvement in the consenting process, this additional information may affect the quoted percentage rates of risks of surgery, such as dead ear in the presence of a fistula. One could argue that patients should have all the potential information regarding the risks of surgery available to them when making an informed choice of treatment.

Cons of CT scanning

The relatively low sensitivity and specificity of CT in identifying abnormalities may lead to surgeons being falsely reassured prior to surgery. As a general rule, it is best practice that all tympanomastoid surgery should be approached with the assumption that there may be an intact ossicular chain, dehiscent facial nerve, and otic capsule fistula. This approach makes CT scanning obsolete. In addition, the dose of radiation associated with CT (especially when multiple fine cuts are obtained) is not insignificant and this has its associated increase in lifetime risk of developing a radiation induced malignancy (although very small). This is probably more relevant in children.

Overall, it is probably fair to say that in the majority of patients a CT scan does not change practice. However, particularly with increasing litigation, some would argue that although only helpful in a small percentage of patients, forewarned is forearmed.

Question 15

A 45-year-old man presents to clinic with hearing loss affecting both ears. See Figures 3.15.1 and 3.15.2.

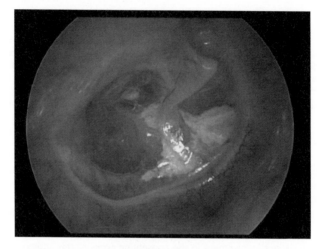

Figure 3.15.1. Right ear.

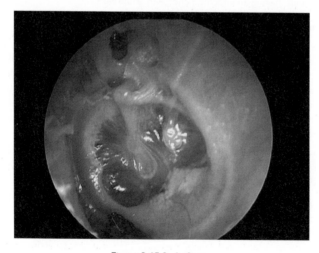

Figure 3.15.2. Left ear.

There is no history of otorrhoea/tinnitus/vertigo. His audiogram is shown in Figure 3.15.3.

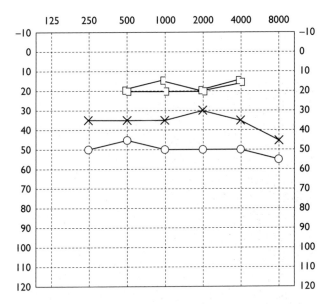

Figure 3.15.3

15.1 Describe the otoendoscopic images.

15.2 Do you know any staging systems for pars tensa and pars flaccida retraction pockets?

15.3 When performing an audiogram, when is masking required?

15.4 When performing an audiogram in this patient what problems may arise with masked bone conduction threshold testing?

15.5 When considering surgery to improve a conductive hearing loss, if you were basing your decision to operate purely on the audiogram, which ear would you operate on?

15.6 Relating to ossiculoplasty, what is the 'Belfast rule of thumb'?

15.7 Can you draw a 'Glasgow benefit plot' and demonstrate which group this patient would be in if operating on the right ear?

Answers to Question 15

15.1 Describe the otoendoscopic images.

The left tympanic membrane has a retraction of the pars tensa onto the incudostapedial joint (ISJ) with probable partial erosion of the long process of the incus (Sade 2). There is a deep retraction of the pars flaccida with erosion of the scutum to expose the malleus head with some keratin on the malleus neck/head suggesting this pocket may not be self-cleaning (Tos 4).

The right tympanic membrane has tympanosclerosis (myringosclerosis) affecting the anteroinferior pars tensa. The posterior pars tensa is retracted onto the head of the stapes (as well as annular retraction). The long process of the incus is absent/eroded.

15.2 Do you know any staging systems for pars tensa and pars flaccida retraction pockets?
- *Sade staging of retractions of pars tensa:*
    1. Mild/annular retraction
    2. Retraction onto ISJ
    3. Retraction onto promontory
    4. Adherent to promontory
- *Tos staging of retractions of pars flaccida:*
    1. Dimple or retraction of pars flaccida, but not in contact with malleus neck
    2. Retraction onto malleus neck
    3. Erosion of scutum
    4. Pocket with keratin/non-self-cleaning (cholesteatoma).

15.3 When performing an audiogram, when is masking required?

Masking of the non-test ear required when testing air conduction (AC) thresholds if:
- >40dB difference in air conduction (AC) thresholds between test and non-test ear
- Difference between poorer hearing ear AC thresholds, and better hearing (non-test) ear bone conduction thresholds, is >40dB
- Masking of bone conduction thresholds is always required if there is a conductive loss (air-bone gap >10dB).

When performing an audiogram, when is masking required?

Rule 1—if there is >40dB difference in AC thresholds between the test and non-test ear
Rule 2—when testing BC thresholds if there is a >10dB air bone gap
Rule 3—if the test ear AC threshold is >40dB worse than the BC in the non-test/better hearing ear.

15.4 When performing an audiogram in this patient what problems may arise with masked bone conduction threshold testing?

The masking dilemma may occur with bilateral conductive hearing loss where adequate intensity to mask the non-test ear crosses over to the testing ear and invalidates the thresholds.

15.5 When considering surgery to improve a conductive hearing loss, if you were basing your decision to operate purely on the audiogram, which ear would you operate on?

The right ear. Although surgery to the left ear may be indicated on the basis of a non-cleaning retraction pocket, audiologically, the right ear is the worse hearing ear.

15.6 Relating to ossiculoplasty, what is the 'Belfast rule of thumb'?

This states that if the operated ear AC threshold is better than 30dBHL, or improved to within 15dB of the better hearing ear, the patient will derive significant benefit from the surgery.

15.7 Can you draw a 'Glasgow benefit plot' and demonstrate which group this patient would be in if operating on the right ear?

This patient has an asymmetrical bilateral hearing loss with an average loss in the better hearing ear of 35dB and 50dB in the worse hearing ear (to be operated). This patient is marked on the plot with an X putting them in group 6; see Figure 3.15.4.

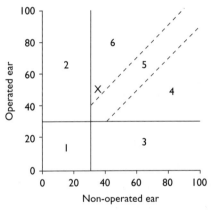

Figure 3.15.4

Question 16

16.1 Please describe the abnormalities seen in the CT shown in Figure 3.16.1.

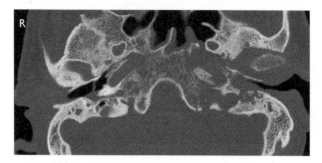

Figure 3.16.1

16.2 What is the most likely diagnosis and what are the differential diagnoses?

16.3 What are the risk factors for this condition?

16.4 What is the most likely pathogen?

16.5 What is the initial route of spread of infection in the pathogenesis of this condition?

16.6 What are the presenting features on history and examination?

16.7 What other investigations would you consider to help confirm your diagnosis?

16.8 What is the role of surgery in the management of this condition?

16.9 How should this patient be treated?

16.10 How can response to treatment be monitored?

16.11 Do you know of any additional treatment modalities used in cases refractory to medical treatment?

Answers to Question 16

16.1 Please describe the abnormalities seen in the CT shown in Figure 3.16.1.

On the left there is soft tissue filling the middle ear and medial external canal, with erosion of the posterior ear canal wall. There is also erosion of the clivus, jugular bulb, and foramen lacerum.

16.2 What is the most likely diagnosis and what are the differential diagnoses?

Skull base osteomyelitis (synonyms—necrotizing otitis externa, malignant otitis externa). Skull base malignancy, Langerhan's cell histiocytosis, granulomatous conditions, bone disorders (Pagets/fibrous dysplasia).

16.3 What are the risk factors for this condition?

Age, diabetes mellitus, immunosuppression. (Also more common in men.)

16.4 What is the most likely pathogen?

Pseudomonas aeroginosa, but rarely can be due to *Staphylococcus aureus*, *Aspergillus* and *Proteus* species.

16.5 What is the initial route of spread of infection in the pathogenesis of this condition?

Otitis externa spreading through the floor of the ear canal through the fissures of Santorini at the bony-cartilaginous junction.

16.6 What are the presenting features on history and examination?

Otorrhoea or a history of otitis externa, severe persistent deep otalgia, hearing loss, lower cranial neuropathies (VII–XII). On examination, there may be evidence of otitis externa with granulation tissue in the floor of the ear canal. Sometimes, even in the presence of continuing skull base osteomyelitis, the ear examination may be unremarkable if the otitis externa has been treated.

16.7 What other investigations would you consider to help confirm your diagnosis?

Blood tests to include FBC, C-reactive protein (CRP)/erythrocyte sedimentation rate (ESR). Swab any ear discharge and send samples for microbiology. Biopsy of ear canal granulation may be possible in clinic. Consider MRI in addition to CT as CT may fail to identify early bone erosion. Less commonly, nuclear imaging techniques are used such as gallium-67 scintigraphy, indium-111 white blood cell scan, technetium-99 bone scan, and single photo emission computed tomography (SPECT). These may be helpful in monitoring response to treatment as MRI/CT findings may persist for up to 6 months following successful treatment.

16.8 What is the role of surgery in the management of this condition?

In general, surgery does not play a significant role in managing this condition as the diagnosis can usually be made clinically. Surgery may be helpful for sampling to obtain tissue for culture to best guide antibiotic/antifungal treatment. In addition, biopsy is helpful to exclude malignancy particularly if the presentation is atypical.

16.9 How should this patient be treated?

Treatment involves aggressive systemic antimicrobial treatment in combination with regular aural toilet and topical antimicrobials. Many patients will be admitted initially for urgent assessment and treatment with intravenous (antipseudomonal) antibiotics. Diabetic patients should have the blood glucose carefully monitored and optimized. Anitmicrobial therapy should be discussed with a microbiologist, but is likely to be prolonged (e.g. 6–12 weeks).

Management of cranial neuropathies may also be required (e.g. eye care in facial nerve palsy or swallow assessment with IX and X involvement).

16.10 How can response to treatment be monitored?

Resolution (or recurrence) of otalgia can be very helpful in conjunction with serial inflammatory markers (white cell count (WCC)/CRP/ESR) and imaging findings.

16.11 Do you know of any additional treatment modalities used in cases refractory to medical treatment?

- Surgical debridement—rare
- Hyperbaric oxygen—expensive.

Question 17

A 46-year-old lady presents 2 weeks following a viral illness, with a 24-h history of rapidly progressive right-sided facial weakness associated with mild right otalgia and hyperacusis to loud noises, such as doors slamming. Initial examination shows normal tone and symmetry at rest, but gross asymmetry on movement with incomplete eye closure and minimal forehead movement on maximum effort.

17.1 How would you grade her weakness using the House–Brackmann classification system?

17.2 What would you look for on examination?

17.3 List common causes of lower motor neuron facial nerve palsy?

17.4 If her examination is otherwise normal, what is the most likely diagnosis and why does why does she have hyperacusis?

17.5 How would you treat this patient?

17.6 How can the facial nerve be tested clinically?

17.7 When should facial nerve electrophysiological testing be performed?

17.8 How can the facial nerve be tested electrophysiologically?

17.9 What are the potential advantages of electrophysiological testing of the facial nerve?

Answers to Question 17

17.1 How would you grade her weakness using the House–Brackmann classification system?

HB IV.

17.2 What would you look for on examination?

Careful facial nerve examination to ensure LMN palsy. Full cranial nerve examination (especially corneal reflex for cranial nerve five (trigeminal nerve; CN V). Ear examination to assess for vesicles, middle ear pathology (cholesteatoma/CSOM), Hitselberger sign. Parotid/neck examination to exclude neoplasm. Oral cavity to assess for palatal weakness, vesicles or parapharyngeal mass. Tuning fork tests to assess hearing, and ideally a formal audiogram.

17.3 List common causes of lower motor neuron facial nerve palsy?

Numerous causes, including those shown in Table 3.17.1.

Acquired	Congenital
Idiopathic/Bell's 50–60%	CHARGE
Viral:	Mobius syndrome
-Ramsay Hunt Syndrome ~10%	Melkersson–Rosenthal syndrome
Bacterial:	Birth trauma/forceps
-Malignant otitis externa	
-Acute otitis media/CSOM	
-Lyme disease	
Traumatic:	
-*Surgical*—parotid, otological, skull base	
-Temporal bone fracture	
Neoplastic:	
-Parotid/glomus/acoustic	
Autoimmune/systemic:	
-Sarcoidosis	
Neurological:	
-Multiple sclerosis/Guillain–Barre	

Table 3.17.1 Common causes of lower motor neuron facial nerve palsy

17.4 If her examination is otherwise normal, what is the most likely diagnosis and why does why does she have hyperacusis?

Idiopathic-sided facial palsy; Bell's palsy. Hyperacusis due to involvement of VII nerve branch to stapedius causing impairment of stapedial reflex.

17.5 How would you treat this patient?

- *Eye care*—ophthalmology review to assess for corneal abrasion/ulceration
  - ◆ Artificial tears/eye drops
  - ◆ Tape eye closed at night
- Medical treatment
- High dose oral steroids (prednisolone) for 7–10 days
- Antivirals advocated in the past, but this is controversial. (They are, however, indicated if vesicles are seen as in Ramsay Hunt syndrome.)

- Exercises to rehabilitate facial muscles
- Review to ensure complete recovery and investigate/imaging if persisting weakness or unusual features.

17.6 How can the facial nerve be tested clinically?

- Facial movement (e.g. grading with House-Brackmann)
- Schirmer's test for lacrimation. Abnormal suggests lesion affecting geniculate ganglion although not very accurate for localization
- Stapedial reflex. Abnormal suggests lesion proximal to nerve to stapedius
- Taste testing either clinically (salt, sweet, sour, bitter) or with electrogustometry and salivary flow testing. If abnormal suggest lesion proximal to root of chorda tympani.

17.7 When should facial nerve electrophysiological testing be performed?

Electrophysiological testing is an indirect assessment of the severity of injury to the intratemporal facial nerve (as this nerve is inaccessible unless stimulated directly intra-operatively). It relies on the fact that a proximal nerve injury will lead to distal Wallerian degeneration and subsequent impairment of distal nerve conduction. As this degeneration usually takes 2–3 days, testing the nerve in the first 1–2 days after injury may lead to a falsely normal result. In addition, after 2–3 weeks, as the nerve begins to recover, there may be asynchronous discharge leading to unreliability in interpreting results. Therefore, testing is most helpful after 2–3 days and up to 2–3 weeks post-injury (often on the 10th day).

17.8 How can the facial nerve be tested electrophysiologically?

Nerve excitability testing

- *Minimal nerve excitability test*—transcutaneous electrodes at stylomastoid foramen on both sides comparing minimum threshold required to produce facial twitch. Difference >3.5mA significant. Subjective—rarely used
- *Maximum stimulation test*—also rarely used as subjective.

Electroneurography

Transcutaneous stimulating electrode at stylomastoid foramen with a measuring surface electrode in the nasolabial fold. Essentially, an evoked electromyography (EMG) comparing normal with injured side. An evoked compound muscle action potential (CAMP) of at least 10% compared with the normal side corresponds to <90% degeneration and a high likelihood of complete recovery. A CAMP of <10% compared with the normal side suggests >90% degeneration and predicts a poorer outcome with increased chance of incomplete facial nerve recovery. (One way to remember this is if <10% response on the 10th day, there is <10% chance of complete recovery). Some surgeons would advocate surgical decompression of the facial nerve in this scenario, but this is controversial.

Electromyography

- This requires needle electrodes to be inserted into the facial muscles and activity is measured during voluntary facial contraction
- This test must be performed after 2 weeks and may show re-innervation potential 4–12 weeks before clinical improvement is noticed.

17.9 What are the potential advantages of electrophysiological testing of the facial nerve?

Electrophysiological studies are quite labour-intensive and require specialist equipment and are not therefore always used routinely, especially when the chance of complete recovery is very high as in this case. They can, however, be useful for prognostication when counselling a patient and, as discussed, they may be helpful in selecting patients who might benefit from facial nerve decompression.

Question 18

A 60-year-old male presents with hearing loss and the audiogram shown in Figure 3.18.1.

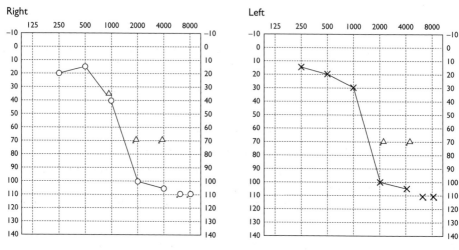

Right   Left

Figure 3.18.1

18.1 Please describe the audiogram in Figure 3.18.1.

18.2 What are the potential aetiologies?

18.3 What other tests are important in assessing this patients hearing disability?

18.4 What are the potential treatment options for this patient?

18.5 What are the audiological criteria for cochlear implantation in adults in the UK?

18.6 What are the basic components of a cochlear implant (CI)?

18.7 Is the low frequency residual hearing a contraindication to CI surgery?

18.8 What are the contraindications to CI surgery?

18.9 If a patient who has a cochlear implant requires surgery for an unrelated condition, what precautions should be taken?

Answers to Question 18

18.1 Please describe the audiogram in Figure 3.18.1.

This audiogram shows bilateral profound hearing loss with a ski-slope pattern with preservation of the lower frequencies.

18.2 What are the potential aetiologies?

Idiopathic sensori-neural deafness (this severity of loss with often have a congenital component), noise-induced hearing loss, ototoxicity-induced hearing loss, mitochondrial gentamicin sensitivity.

18.3 What other tests are important in assessing this patients hearing disability?

Speech audiogram/speech discrimination scores.

18.4 What are the potential treatment options for this patient?

The two main options to help rehabilitate this patients hearing loss are:

- *Hearing aid trial*—patients with this pattern of hearing loss often do not derive great benefit from conventional hearing aids, but frequency shifting hearing aids can be helpful
- *Cochlear implantation*—if the patient's hearing loss cannot be helped with conventional hearing aids.

18.5 What are the audiological criteria for cochlear implantation in adults in the UK?

NICE guidance 2009 for adults

Unilateral cochlear implantation is recommended as an option for people with severe to profound deafness who do not receive adequate benefit from acoustic hearing aids. For this purpose, severe/profound hearing loss is defined as hearing thresholds of worse than 90dB at 2 and 4 kHz. Inadequate benefit from hearing aids is defined as scores of <50% on Bamford–Kowal–Bench (BKB) sentence testing at a sound intensity of 70dB sound pressure level (SPL) in best aided conditions.

18.6 What are the basic components of a cochlear implant (CI)?

External component

Microphone, sound processor, transmitter coil.

Internal component

Induction coil and magnet, receiver/stimulator, electrode array.

18.7 Is the low frequency residual hearing a contraindication to CI surgery?

No. Although residual low frequency hearing may be damaged or lost with the insertion of a CI, these lower frequencies (<1kHz) do not contribute significantly to speech discrimination. However, it may be possible to preserve these lower frequencies with the use of a hybrid electrode and 'soft surgery'. This would have the advantage for improved sound localization, binaural listening, and music perception.

18.8 What are the contraindications to CI surgery?

Absolute

Absent cochlear nerve/central deafness, completely ossified cochlea.

Relative

- *CSOM, mastoid cavity*—should be treated/obliterated first
- Longstanding profound hearing loss, especially if prelingually deaf and never aided. Very poor candidates as unlikely to derive significant benefit
- Not medically fit for surgery.

18.9 If a patient who has a cochlear implant requires surgery for an unrelated condition, what precautions should be taken?

Prior to surgery the external sound processor should be removed. Monopolar diathermy should be avoided. Bipolar may be used, but not close to the device.

Further reading

National Institute for Health and Clinical Excellence (2009). *Cochlear implants for severe to profound deafness in children and adults*, Technology appraisals TA166. London: NICE. Available at: http://www.nice.org.uk/TA166

Question 19

19.1   What device is shown in Figures 3.19.1 and 3.19.2?

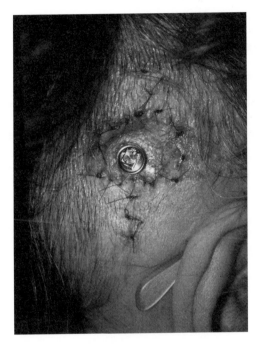

Figure 3.19.1

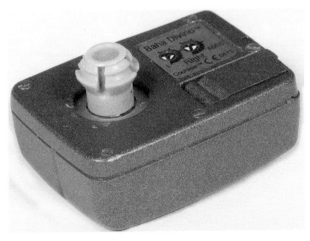

Figure 3.19.2

19.2   What are the indications?

19.3   What are the contraindications?

19.4   What are the components of this device?

19.5   What material is the implanted component made of and why?

19.6   How would you assess a patient's suitability for this device pre-operatively?

19.7   From what age can this device be used?

19.8   What are the complications of this surgery?

19.9   When can the abutment be loaded?

19.10   The patient is likely to require MRI scanning in the future, what should you tell them?

19.11   What would be an alternative hearing aid to use in single-sided deafness?

Answers to Question 19

19.1 What device is shown in Figures 3.19.1 and 3.19.2?

Bone anchored hearing aid.

19.2 What are the indications?

Conductive hearing loss (bilateral/unilateral), but unable use conventional air conduction hearing aid due to:

- Congenital ear canal atresia or acquired meatal stenosis or very narrow ear canals (e.g. Down's syndrome)
- CSOM/discharging mastoid cavity
- Recurrent or chronic otitis externa, where wearing hearing aid exacerbates condition
- Single sided deafness (sensori-neural).

19.3 What are the contraindications?

Audiological

- Cochlear thresholds (SNHL) worse than 55dB in better hearing ear
- Poor speech discrimination (<60%).

Surgical

- Skin conditions affecting implant area—psoriasis, eczema, infections.
- Bone conditions: Osteogenesis imperfect, Pagets.

19.4 What are the components of this device?

- Fixture, which is a titanium screw
- Abutment
- External sound processor, consisting of microphone, digital processor, and vibrating component with a snap fit coupling to the abutment.

19.5 What material is the implanted component made of and why?

Pure titanium, which has the property of osseointegration.

19.6 How would you assess a patient's suitability for this device pre-operatively?

PTA with masked bone conduction thresholds, then trial of a soft band bone conducting aid. Patients who derive significant benefit from this trial are likely to be good candidates for a bone-anchored hearing aid (BAHA).

19.7 From what age can this device be used?

Most surgeons wait until at least 5 years of age to ensure adequate skull thickness but in specialist centres as young as 18 months.

19.8 What are the complications of this surgery?

- *Early*—skin flap haematoma, infection, necrosis
- *Late*—failure of osseointegration, loosening, trauma, skin overgrowth/infection.

19.9 When can the abutment be loaded?

Conventionally, this was delayed until 3 months post-implantation to ensure adequate osseointegration. However, some newer designs are being loaded much earlier.

19.10 The patient is likely to require MRI scanning in the future, what should you tell them?

The fixture and abutment are made of titanium and are non-ferrous, and are therefore safe for MRI scanning. The sound processor **does** contain ferrous components and must therefore be removed. The fixture and abutment may, however, cause artefact when imaging the brain.

19.11 What would be an alternative hearing aid to use in single-sided deafness?

A contralateral routing of signal (CROS) aid would be a good alternative.

Question 20

A 60-year-old businessman presents to clinic complaining of hearing loss and tinnitus. His hearing loss is worse in background noise and his tinnitus is bilateral and high-pitched. Neuro-otological examination is normal. His audiogram is shown in Figure 3.20.1.

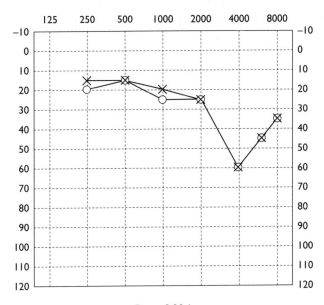

Figure 3.20.1

20.1 What does his audiogram show and what is the likely diagnosis?

20.2 How would you manage this patient?

20.3 What are the basic components of a hearing aid?

20.4 What different styles of hearing aid are seen in Figure 3.20.2a–e and what are their relative advantages?

20.5 Which would be an appropriate initial option for this patient?

20.6 What is dynamic range and how is it affected by presbyacusis?

20.7 How do digital hearing aids help with these changes?

20.8 Would you offer this patient one hearing aid or two and why?

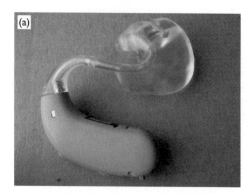

Figure 3.20.2a

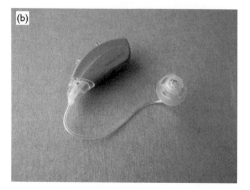

Figure 3.20.2b

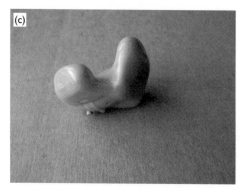

Figure 3.20.2c

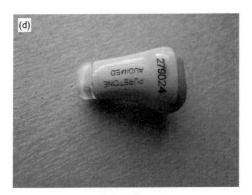

Figure 3.20.2d

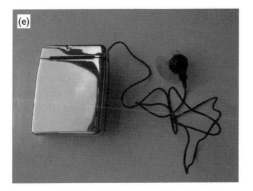

Figure 3.20.2e

Answers to Question 20

20.1 What does his audiogram show and what is the likely diagnosis?

Pure tone audiogram showing high frequency SNHL bilaterally consistent with presbyacusis.

20.2 How would you manage this patient?

Management largely tailored to patient's needs:

> Patient education, offer hearing aid to treat hearing loss and tinnitus, reassurance regarding tinnitus +/– tinnitus therapy/counselling.

20.3 What are the basic components of a hearing aid?

Microphone, amplifier, sound transmitter/speaker, power source.

20.4 What different styles of hearing aid are seen in Figure 3.20.2a–e and what are their relative advantages?

Most modern hearing aids are digital (rather than analogue) and the type usually refers to the size or physical appearance/design of the aid. These include those listed in Table 3.20.1.

Type of HA	Advantages/indications	Disadvantage
Behind-the-ear (BTE), with custom mould (Fig 3.20.2a)	Most commonly used as good for the majority of patients as can accommodate wide range of hearing losses	Tight fitting/non-vented moulds may be required to prevent feedback, especially if severe/profound loss. This can predispose to humidity with otitis externa/ear infections
BTE with open fit mould (Fig 3.20.2b)	Can be fitted at one sitting as no custom mould required. Open fit provides excellent ventilation to reduce the occlusion effect and reduce humidity. Cosmesis.	Indication limited to mild and moderate loss. Feedback
In-the-ear/In-the-canal/completely-in-the-canal ITE/ITC/CIC (Fig 3.20.2c and d)	Less obvious or even unnoticeable. Easier to insert/remove.	Feedback more likely as microphone closer to speaker Expensive More likely to malfunction from cerumen impaction requiring repair Unsuitable for children as must be resized with growth
Body worn (Fig 3.20.2e)	Powerful, good for profound loss. Feedback rarely a problem. Good if poor manual dexterity.	Cosmetic May pick up unwanted noises such as clothes rubbing

Table 3.20.1 Types of modern hearing aid

20.5 Which would be an appropriate initial option for this patient?

A behind the ear hearing aid with an open fit mould would be appropriate.

20.6 What is dynamic range and how is it affected by presbyacusis?

Dynamic range (DR) is the difference between the threshold for hearing and the loudness discomfort level (for a given test frequency). In a normal ear, this is around 100dB. In cochlear hearing loss, hearing threshold increases, thereby reducing the dynamic range. As a result, in this group, a small increase in sound intensity may be perceived as disproportionately and uncomfortably large increase in loudness; this is known as recruitment. The exact physiological mechanism for loudness recruitment is yet to be fully understood.

20.7 How do digital hearing aids help with these changes?

Digital hearing aids have the advantage of superior signal processing which allow for signal *compression*. That is, they can be programmed to ensure the output does not exceed the patient's loudness discomfort levels. Historically, analogue hearing aids could have their output limited either with a gain control, or by 'clipping' the amplitude peaks, which produces distortion.

20.8 Would you offer this patient one hearing aid or two and why?

Patients with bilateral symmetrical hearing loss should always be offered two hearing aids as there are some clear advantages:

- Improved sound localization
- Binaural summation means that hearing with both ears can improve loudness by up to 6dB, reducing gain requirements thereby potentially reducing feedback problems
- Binaural squelch is the improved ability to listen to the sound source of interest in the presence of background noise. Monaural hearing reduces the listener's ability to use sound localization clues and, therefore, requires a greater signal-to-noise ratio.

Chapter 4

Paediatrics

Question 1

1.1 What are the otoscopic findings in acute otitis media?

1.2 What is the definition of acute otitis media?

1.3 What are the risk factors for developing acute otitis media?

1.4 What are the most common organisms implicated in the development of the condition?

1.5 How would you go about managing the condition?

1.6 What are the possible complications associated with acute otitis media?

1.7 What options are available in managing children with recurrent episodes of acute otitis media?

Answers to Question 1

1.1 What are the otoscopic findings in acute otitis media?

A bulging erythematous tympanic membrane and middle ear fluid.

1.2 What is the definition of acute otitis media?

- Acute suppurative otitis media is the presence of a purulent effusion in the middle ear cleft associated with systemic signs and symptoms of infection
- Most common age of presentation is 3 months to 3 years. By age 3, 50–85% have had at least one episode.

1.3 What are the risk factors for developing acute otitis media?

Risk factors can be divided into host and environmental.

Host

- Age <6 months
- Male
- Underlying predisposing factors- cleft palate, craniofacial abnormalities, Eustachian tube dysfunction, barotraumas, cochlear implantation, immune deficiencies, Down's syndrome
- Very low birth weight/preterm <33 weeks
- Possibly reflux, but this is controversial.

Environmental

- *Seasonal*—increase in autumn/winter
- Day care/multiple siblings
- Passive smoking
- Low socio-economic group
- Use of dummy.

1.4 What are the most common organisms implicated in the development of the condition?

Bacterial

- *Strep pneumoniae*
- *Haemophilus influenzae*
- *Moraxella catarrhalis*
- Less commonly—anaerobes and *Pseudomonas aeruginosa*.

Viral

- Respiratory syncytial virus
- Influenza virus (type A or B)
- Adenovirus.

1.5 How would you go about managing the condition?

Confirm diagnosis from history and otoscopic examination. Treat with antipyretic/analgesics. The role of antibiotics is controversial as the condition is often self-limiting. However, if antibiotics are not prescribed, medical follow-up is advisable. The presence of the following factors, which increase the risk of complications, would prompt most to treat with antibiotics:

- Age <2
- Recurrent AOM
- Severe clinical symptoms
- Underlying immune deficiency.

In an uncomplicated infection in an older child many would wait and watch for the first 48–72h and treat only if significant symptoms persist beyond this period. Evidence suggests antibiotics have a small impact upon the duration of pain.

1.6 What are the possible complications associated with acute otitis media?

Intratemporal

Tympanic membrane perforation, acute mastoiditis, facial paralysis, subperiosteal abscess, Bezold/Citelli's abscesses, labyrinthitis—SNHL and vertigo.

Intracranial

Meningitis, lateral sinus thrombosis, brain abscess, otitic hydrocephalus

1.7 What options are available in managing children with recurrent episodes of acute otitis media?

- A period of 2–3 months of once daily prophylactic antibiotics, such as amoxicillin
- *Grommet insertion*—Burton *et al.* (2011) shows evidence of reduction in episodes after grommet insertion, though evidence is limited.

Further reading

Burton MJ, Derkay CS, Rosenfeld RM (2011). Extracts from The Cochrane Library: 'Grommets (ventilation tubes) for hearing loss associated with otitis media with effusion in children'. *Otolaryngol Head Neck Surg* **144**(2): 657–61.

Question 2

In recent months, the child shown in Figure 4.2.1 has had mucinous discharge from the point marked.

2.1 What does Figure 4.2.1 show?

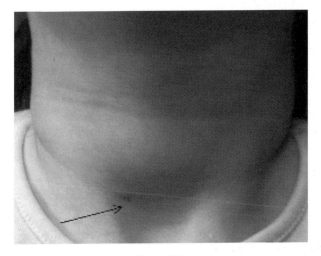

Figure 4.2.1

2.2 What is the embryological origin of this and what anatomical course do you expect it to run?

2.3 How would you manage this patient?

2.4 What are the key steps in the surgical approach?

2.5 What other branchial cleft anomalies do you know and how do these present?

2.6 How would you manage them?

2.7 Which are the most and least common branchial anomalies?

Answers to Question 2

2.1 What does Figure 4.2.1 show?

A photograph of a child's neck with an infected sinus mid-lower neck at the anterior border of sternocleidomastoid muscle.

2.2 What is the embryological origin of this and what anatomical course do you expect it to run?

This is the typical appearance of a second branchial cleft sinus/fistula. It runs from the sinus opening in the neck superiorly along the carotid sheath, anterior to the hypoglossal nerve and deep to the posterior belly of digastric, passing between the internal and external carotid arteries, and extending towards/opening into the ipsilateral tonsillar fossa.

2.3 How would you manage this patient?

The majority of patients present by the age of 5 years. They may be asymptomatic, or have recurring pain and discharge from the sinus opening. Some surgeons would arrange a sinogram to delineate the tract, but others feel it unnecessary and proceed to surgical excision without investigations.

2.4 What are the key steps in the surgical approach?

Methylene blue injection or use of a lacrimal probe can help identify the tract. Elliptical incision to remove sinus opening. Identify and follow the tract superiorly. This is not a branching tract; therefore, there is no need to excise any surrounding tissue, staying close onto the tract reduces the chance of damaging nearby neurovascular structures. The tract is followed superiorly until it ends or passes into the pharyngeal musculature. In young children this can be achieved through a single incision. In older children/adolescents it may require a stepladder type approach with a further incision superiorly. At this point options are to tie and divide it at this level or follow it into the oropharynx with removal of the ipsilateral tonsil.

2.5 What other branchial cleft anomalies do you know and how do these present?

1st cleft

Presentation—2 main subtypes: tract 1 runs from auricular area parallel to external canal; tract 2 runs from skin of anterior neck above the hyoid along the border of the body of mandible with tract coursing superiorly over the mandible through the parotid towards the bony/cartilaginous junction of the ear canal. Presentation therefore varies from a peri-auricular sinus or abscess, external canal swelling or discharge, and/or an abscess or sinus opening along the line of the mandible. Always examine the ear canal. There are three accepted classifications of which the one by Work is most frequently used, whereby type one is one that includes ectodermal tissue only whereas type two is on which includes both ectodermal and mesodermal tissue. However it does not help the surgeon with the surgical relationship to the facial nerve. The classification by Olsen is perhaps the most useful, where type one is a cyst, type two is a sinus, and type three is a fistula.

3rd/4th cleft

Presentation—tract runs inferiorly from piriform fossa into the neck with no external opening and usually presents in child or early adulthood with either recurrent thyroiditis or anterior neck abscesses.

2.6 How would you manage them?

1st cleft

Imaging is helpful to define the anatomy and possibly the relationship to the facial nerve. Sinogram/CT/MRI. Surgery requires a parotidectomy approach to protect the facial nerve, and complete excision of the tract.

3rd/4th cleft

Barium swallow demonstrates the tract extending inferiorly from the piriform fossa. Surgical excision of the tract +/− hemithyroidectomy has been the treatment of choice until recently when an endoscopic approach with diathermy/tissue glue closure of the sinus opening in the piriform fossa has been shown to be successful and avoided the need for open surgery.

2.7 Which are the most and least common branchial anomalies?

- *2nd cleft*—>90% (it should be noted that 'branchial cysts' typically present in early adulthood and their pathogenesis is often challenged as to whether they are truly branchiogenic or whether they represent epithelial rests or degeneration within a lymph node)
- *1st cleft*—8%
- *3/4th cleft*—<2%.

Question 3

3.1 What is the scan shown in Figure 4.3.1 and what does it reveal?

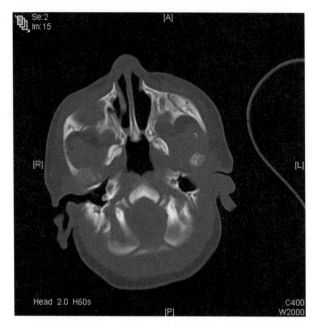

Figure 4.3.1

3.2 Do you know any pathophysiological theories to explain the abnormality?

3.3 How and when would you expect this patient to present?

3.4 How would that differ if it were uni/bilateral?

3.5 What are the initial steps in management?

3.6 Are you aware of any associations and how might you assess the presence of these?

3.7 Briefly describe the surgical approach to treating the condition.

Answers to Question 3

3.1 What is the scan shown in Figure 4.3.1 and what does it reveal?

This is an axial CT scan of the nose and para-nasal sinuses on bone window settings showing soft tissue/bony occlusion of posterior nasal cavity suggestive of choanal atresia. The CT scan can demonstrate whether a choanal atresia is bony, membranous or mixed. This has ramifications for the surgical approach.

3.2 Do you know any pathophysiological theories to explain the abnormality?

Several have been described including:
- Persistence of the buccopharyngeal membrane
- Failure of rupture of the bucconasal membrane
- Formation of mesodermal adhesions in the choana
- Overgrowth of vertical and horizontal processes of the palatine bone medially.

3.3 How and when would you expect this patient to present?

Typically within the first few days of life with respiratory distress and cyanotic episodes—especially on feeding, relieved by crying. This is due to the fact that neonates are predominantly obligate nasal breathers until around 3 months of age. Sometimes, the suspicion is raised by an inability to pass a nasogastric tube or a suction catheter through the nostril.

3.4 How would that differ if it were uni/bilateral?

Unilateral atresia is much less likely to present early unless there were a failed attempt to pass an NGT. More commonly presents with unilateral purulent rhinorrhea/congestion in an older child.

3.5 What are the initial steps in management?

Oral airway, modified teat or McGovern nipple taped in. Avoid intubation if possible. Transfer to paediatric centre for definitive management

3.6 Are you aware of any associations and how might you assess the presence of these?

Bilateral choanal atresia is commonly part of a polymalformation syndrome.

CHARGE syndrome is the most common

C—coloboma

H—heart defects

A—atresia choanae

R—retardation of growth and/or development

G—genitourinary abnormalities

E—ear abnormalities/deafness.

Review by general paediatrician +/− cardiology, ophthalmology, endocrinology. It is particularly important to assess for the presence of serious cardiac anomalies before proceeding with surgery.

3.7 Briefly describe the surgical approach to treating the condition.

The classical transpalatal approach has largely been superseded by endoscopic/intranasal surgery. Two main variations are passage of both endoscope and instruments intranasally contrasting with use of a 120-degree endoscope passed intraorally to visualize the posterior choana together with intranasal instruments. The nose is prepared with decongestants, a mucosal flap may be raised, then various tools have been described to open the choana—CO_2 and KTP lasers, cutting/diamond burrs, and urethral sounds. It is common practice to also remove the posterior vomer. Attempts to reduce the risk of restenosis with topical mitomycin C and the use of stents are also described.

Question 4

A 4-year-old boy presents to the Emergency Department with a three day history of a swollen right eye. Clinically, this looks like peri-orbital cellulitis.

4.1 What is the usual clinical scenario in these circumstances?

4.2 What is the commonest cause, and differential diagnosis?

4.3 What are the key features you would look for on examination?

4.4 Do you know any staging systems used for this condition?

4.5 What is the orbital septum?

4.6 How would you manage the patient?

4.7 What are the surgical options?

Answers to Question 4

4.1 What is the usual clinical scenario in these circumstances?

Preceding symptoms of an upper respiratory tract infection, particularly nasal obstruction, and rhinor-rhoea. Following this, the development of peri-orbital erythema, swelling, and tenderness.

4.2 What is the commonest cause, and differential diagnosis?

The most common is secondary to spread of infection from acute ethmoid sinusitis, with main organisms: *Streptococcus pneumoniae*, *Haemophilus influenza*, and *Staphyloccocus aureus*.

Differential

Primary skin/soft tissue infection associated with local trauma/insect bite, dacrocystitis.

4.3 What are the key features you would look for on examination?

General status of the child from a neurological point of view. Examine the nose for evidence of acute inflammation and purulent secretions. Examine the eyes—opening, pupillary reflexes, colour vision, acuity, eye movements, proptosis, chemosis.

4.4 Do you know any staging systems used for this condition?

Staging

Chandler (1970, see Box 4.4.1): the disease process does not necessarily follow a step wise progression.

Box 4.4.1 Chandler's classification

I Pre-septal
II Post-septal without abscess
III Subperiosteal abscess
IV Orbital abscess
V Cavernous sinus thrombosis.

Reproduced from 'The pathogenesis of orbital complications in acute sinusitis', James R. Chandler, David J. Langenbrunner, Edward R. Stevens,. *The Laryngoscope* **80**(9): 1414–28. copyright 2009 with permission of John Wiley and Sons.

The presence of eye signs suggests progression beyond stage 1.

4.5 What is the orbital septum?

The orbital septum acts as a barrier to the spread of infection from skin and subcutaneous tissues into the orbit. It is a fibrous membrane that lies just deep to the orbicularis oculi muscle extending from the periosteum of the orbit to the levator aponeurosis in the upper eyelid and to the inferior border of the tarsal plate in the lower eyelid.

4.6 How would you manage the patient?

Admit. Paediatric and ophthalmology reviews same day. HR/temp, orbital, and neurological observations frequently (hourly). Full blood count, inflammatory markers, and blood cultures. Nasal swabs frequently unhelpful. Broad spectrum IV antibiotics, topical +/− systemic decongestants.

Indications for CT: (consider MRI for cavernous sinus/intracranial spread)

• Failure to improve after 24hrs medical treatment
• Eye signs/unable to adequately assess eye
• Deterioration in condition
• Bilateral symptoms.

If a sub-periosteal abscess is confirmed on CT many would suggest that surgical drainage is mandatory. However, in a well child with no adverse orbital signs others would continue conservative treatment and close observation, with evidence suggesting a proportion will resolve without the need for surgery.

4.7 What are the surgical options?

Open vs. endoscopic approach—difficulties with the endoscopic approach include limited access due to the young age of the child, and excessive bleeding in an acutely inflamed nasal cavity. Open approach: modified Lynch Howarth/brow incision with notch to prevent webbing; dissection through periosteum to identify the anterior lacrimal crest; sub-periosteal dissection into the orbit until meet abscess cavity; wash out; consider some form of external ethmoidectomy to facilitate ongoing drainage; insert a drain, e.g. Yates/corrugated/catheter for 24–48h; consider at least a maxillary sinus washout. Endoscopic approach also presents a greater risk of frontonasal stenosis.

Further reading

Chandler JR, Langerbrunner DJ, Stevens ER (2009). The pathogenesis of orbital complications in acute sinusitis. *Laryngoscope* **80**(9): 1414–28.

Question 5

Figure 4.5.1 shows a left tympanic membrane, fluid in the middle ear cleft and no inflammation.

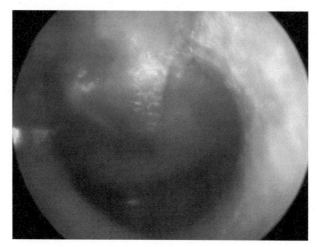

Figure 4.5.1

5.1 What age is the peak incidence?

5.2 What are the risk factors?

5.3 What are the key points to ask in the history?

5.4 How do you manage this condition?

5.5 What differs in the management of otitis media with effusion in children with cleft palate?

5.6 What are your main considerations in deciding whether to perform a myringoplasty in a child with a persisting perforation 12 months after extrusion of a grommet?

Answers to Question 5

5.1 What age is the peak incidence?

Bimodal distribution with peaks at 2–3 and 5 years. Usually resolves by 8–10 years.

5.2 What are the risk factors?

- Cleft palate
- Down's syndrome
- Parental smoking
- Children in nursery/day-care
- Siblings with OME
- Bottle fed
- Low socioeconomic group.

5.3 What are the key points to ask in the history?

- What are concerns re hearing, listening skills, behavioural problems?
- Speech and language development
- Educational progress
- Duration of concerns
- Related episodes of acute otitis media
- Symptoms of nasal obstruction and snoring.

5.4 How do you manage this condition?

History as described. Examination—otoscopy, general ENT and development. Age appropriate audiometry, tympanometry.

OME tends to fluctuate and will resolve within 3 months in a significant proportion of cases (20–50%). NICE guidelines (2008) therefore suggest a period of 3 months active observation, with surgical intervention then considered for those with persisting bilateral OME with hearing level 25–30dB in the better hearing ear. Hearing aids should be offered as an alternative to surgery (see Further reading).

5.5 What differs in the management of otitis media with effusion in children with cleft palate?

Children with cleft palate have Eustachian tube dysfunction resulting in an increased risk of otitis media with effusion. This tends to occur earlier in life, persist for longer and recur more frequently therefore requiring multiple surgical interventions with increase in associated complications. It is therefore recommended that hearing aids should be offered as a first line treatment in preference to grommet insertion.

5.6 What are your main considerations in deciding whether to perform a myringoplasty in a child with a persisting perforation 12 months after extrusion of a grommet?

- Age of the child
- Condition of the other ear: persisting evidence of OME/Eustachian tube dysfunction (ETD), hearing.
- Symptoms related to the perforation—recurring infections, difficulties swimming, hearing.

Unless the severity of symptoms relating to the perforation is causing serious concern, most surgeons would advise waiting until clear resolution of OME in the contralateral ear +/− the child reaching the age of 10–12 years.

Further reading

NICE (2008). *Surgical management of children with otitis media with effusion (OME)*, guideline CG60. Available at: http://guidance.nice.org.uk/CG60

Question 6

You are called urgently to the resuscitation area in the Emergency Department to see a 3-year-old child who had a tonsillectomy 8 days ago and is now bleeding.

6.1 How would you initially manage the child?

6.2 What are normal heart rate (HR)/blood pressure (BP)/respiration rate (RR) in a 3-year-old child?

6.3 What is the blood volume of a 15kg child and how much blood can they lose before significant hypovolaemic shock occurs?

6.4 If there is evidence of hypovolaemia, what volume of fluid would you give?

6.5 How would you approach surgical management of the bleeding?

Answers to Question 6

6.1 How would you initially manage the child?

- Rapid assessment of the severity of compromise by conscious level, whether child alert and co-operative, evidence of ongoing active bleeding, capillary refill, and parameters which indicate level of hypovolaemic shock—HR/BP/RR/(urine output)
- History from parents about duration and severity of bleeding up to now, but bear in mind that young children often swallow blood
- IV access, IV fluids if appropriate, Blood tests—FBC, group and save (G+S)/cross-match
- If theatre needed, inform anaesthetist and theatre staff.

6.2 What are normal HR/BP/RR in a 3-year-old child?

- HR 80–130
- BP 90–105/55–70
- RR 20–30.

6.3 What is the blood volume of a 15kg child and how much blood can they lose before significant hypovolaemic shock occurs?

Blood volume in children is calculated as 80ml/kg = 1200ml
- Grade 1 shock = loss of 15% blood volume (180ml)
- Grade 2 shock = 15–30% blood volume (180–360ml)
- Grade 3 shock = 30–40% blood volume (360–480ml)
- Grade 4 shock = 40–50% blood volume (480–600ml).

Children will tend to compensate for longer than adults, i.e. maintain BP despite significant volume losses. They will deteriorate more rapidly once they decompensate; therefore, a high level of suspicion and very close observation is required.

6.4 If there is evidence of hypovolaemia, what volume of fluid would you give?

20ml/kg crystalloid =300ml in this case. This can be repeated one further time dependent on response, but bear in mind that there is a risk of developing pulmonary oedema if volume greater than this is infused rapidly—the child may then require high level care.

6.5 How would you approach surgical management of the bleeding?

Ensure an experienced anaesthetist is present as intubation can be challenging in a bleeding child with a stomach full of blood. Approach as per tonsillectomy with Boyle Davis gag, Draffin rods, etc. Identify bleeding site if possible—use bipolar cautery or ties. If there is no obvious site consider suturing together anterior and posterior pillars +/− surgicel/haemostatic agent. Use a large bore NGT to empty any residual blood from the stomach, both to more accurately assess blood loss and prevent further vomiting peri-operatively.

Question 7

7.1 What does Figure 4.7.1 show?

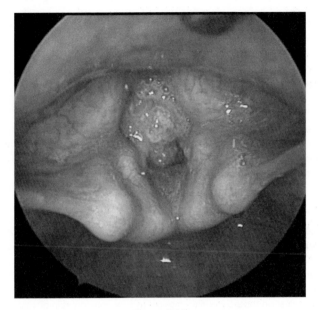

Figure 4.7.1

7.2 At what age does this condition tend to present and with what symptoms?

7.3 What is the aetiology?

7.4 What are the principles of management?

7.5 What is the prognosis?

7.6 Is tracheostomy indicated in this condition?

7.7 Do you know of any adjuvant therapies used?

7.8 What do you know about the HPV vaccination programme in the UK?

Answers to Question 7

7.1 What does Figure 4.7.1 show?

An endoscopic photograph of the larynx taken during surgery showing respiratory papillomata obstructing the glottis.

7.2 At what age does this condition tend to present and with what symptoms?

Age 3–5 is the classic age for children to present. The most common symptom is hoarse voice, and after vocal cord nodules, this is the commonest cause of hoarseness in young children. In more advanced cases there may also be symptoms of airway obstruction, particularly on exertion.

7.3 What is the aetiology?

HPV subtypes 6 and 11 are the primary agents responsible. Transmission is vertical from infected mothers who may have frank viral genital warts (condylomata accuminata). This is felt predominantly to occur during passage through the birth canal and vaginal delivery is a risk factor. However there is no good evidence that Caesarean section prevents transmission. (HPV DNA has been identified in amniotic fluid and umbilical cord blood, which may explain this.)

7.4 What are the principles of management?

Control of symptoms as there is no known cure. Depending on severity this may involve multiple/frequent surgical procedures. This is achieved by microlaryngoscopy and removal of the papillomata with microdebrider/CO_2 or KTP laser/cold steel instruments. A balance must be struck between removal of disease and causing damage to underlying structures with scarring and poor voice outcomes. At least at the first procedure, biopsy should be taken to confirm diagnosis. There is also a very small risk of malignant transformation though in children this is usually only found in disease involving the distal bronchopulmonary tract.

7.5 What is the prognosis?

Difficult to predict at outset. The frequency that procedures are required becomes evident over time, though can be variable and recurrences after long periods of remission have been seen. Evidence suggests at least half of patients with recurrent respiratory papillomatosis (RRP) will require ten or more surgical procedures and 7% over 100. Involvement of the trachea has been reported in a quarter of patients; distal bronchopulmonary involvement is much rarer (5%) and poses greater challenges in management. HPV-11 is associated with a more aggressive phenotype.

7.6 Is tracheostomy indicated in this condition?

Occasionally, if the patient presents with severe obstruction this may be necessary. The consensus is that it should be avoided if possible, and if needed should be reversed as soon as control of the disease is achieved. There is evidence that tracheostomy may increase the risk of distal tracheal spread, though it is not clear if the tracheostomy is causative or simply those children requiring it have more aggressive disease.

7.7 Do you know of any adjuvant therapies used?

There are several agents described. Evidence for their efficacy is limited and they are therefore reserved for those with aggressive disease requiring very frequent surgical intervention. They include cidofovir, indole-3-carbinol, alpha interferon, and photodynamic therapy. There have been recent concerns regarding evidence of *in vitro* up regulation of oncogenes with the use of cidofovir and it must be remembered that the use of cidofovir in this condition is considered 'off-licence' and, therefore, must be authorized on a case-by-case basis by the local institution drugs and therapeutics committee.

7.8 What do you know about the HPV vaccination programme in the UK?

Started in September 2008. Given to teenage girls age 12–13. Coverage in England was 76.4%. The vaccine chosen is bivalent (Cervarix) which only protects against HPV 16 and 18—those implicated in cervical cancer with no protection against genital warts or RRP. As of 2012 in the UK, HPV vaccination will be by the quadrivalent vaccine (Gardasil), which has additional protection against HPV 6 and 11.

Question 8

8.1 What does Figure 4.8.1 show?

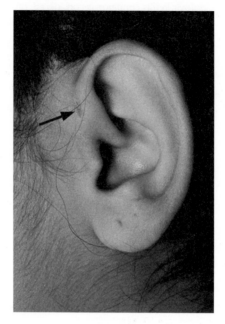

Figure 4.8.1

8.2 What is the embryological origin of this abnormality?

8.3 How is it inherited?

8.4 How does the patient present?

8.5 Are you aware of any associations?

8.6 How would you manage the patient?

8.7 What are the key steps in the surgical approach?

8.8 How common is recurrence following surgery and what factors increase the risk of this occurring?

Answers to Question 8

8.1 What does Figure 4.8.1 show?

A child with a non-infected left pre-auricular sinus.

8.2 What is the embryological origin of this abnormality?

The auricle arises from 1st and 2nd branchial arches during the 6th week of gestation. Each contributes three of the six hillocks of his, which should unite over the following weeks. Pre-auricular sinuses occur as a result of failure of this process. The tract is narrow, may branch and tends to involve at least the perichondrium of the helical/tragal cartilage. The majority are lateral and superior to the facial nerve, though the tract may enter the parotid gland.

8.3 How is it inherited?

Inheritance—incomplete autosomal dominant with reduced penetrance/variable expression.

8.4 How does the patient present?

Often asymptomatic. If symptomatic episodes of discharging tract/abscess/ulceration/facial cellulitis. 25–50% are bilateral

8.5 Are you aware of any associations?

Treacher-Collins sundrome, branchio-oto-renal syndrome, hemifacial microsomia.

8.6 How would you manage the patient?

Conservative if asymptomatic. Once symptomatic it is likely to give further problems with recurring infections; therefore, surgical excision is indicated.

8.7 What are the key steps in the surgical approach?

Use of lacrimal probes/methylene blue to delineate tract is described. The alternative approach is to perform a wide local excision to ensure including all branches of the tract. Elliptical incision; follow tract down to pre-parotid fascia; it is important to excise a small amount of surrounding auricular cartilage together with the tract in order to minimize the risk of recurrence.

8.8 How common is recurrence following surgery and what factors increase the risk of this occurring?

Recurrence rate is reported between 5 and 40%. Risk factors for recurrence include previous infection/abscess drainage, current infection, removal under local anaesthetic, failure to remove cartilage, revision procedure.

Question 9

9.1 What does Figure 4.9.1 show?

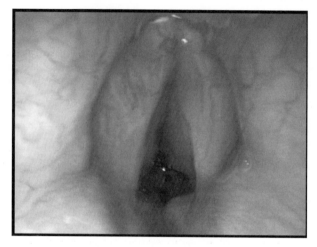

Figure 4.9.1

9.2 What are the main differences between the adult and paediatric larynx?

9.3 What symptoms would a child with this condition present with?

9.4 What are the risk factors/associations with its development?

9.5 Are you aware of any staging systems?

9.6 How is the condition managed?

9.7 What are the main surgical options?

Answers to Question 9

9.1 What does Figure 4.9.1 show?

Endoscopic photo of the larynx showing subglottic stenosis.

9.2 What are the main differences between the adult and paediatric larynx?

- Paediatric larynx is higher (C1–C4), adult C4–C7
- Paediatric larynx is funnel shaped with cricoid its narrowest point, adult larynx glottis is narrowest point
- Paediatric epiglottis is omega shaped and angled away from the trachea
- Paediatric tongue is relatively larger.

9.3 What symptoms would a child with this condition present with?

This will depend on the degree of stenosis. At the mild end of the spectrum episodic croup type episodes with concurrent URTIs and/or mild exertion related breathlessness/stridor. In more severe cases persistent biphasic stridor and respiratory distress at rest may be present.

9.4 What are the risk factors/associations with its development?

It can be congenital or acquired.

- *Congenital*—may be membranous or cartilaginous. Cartilaginous stenoses are generally more severe and are associated with an ovoid cricoid ring. There is an increased incidence in children with Down's syndrome
- *Acquired*—risk factors are prolonged intubation, size of endotracheal tube, repeated re-intubations, low birth weight (<1500g), infection, presence of NGT/reflux, thermal/caustic injuries.

9.5 Are you aware of any staging systems?

The Cotton Classification System is widely used. Staging is usually performed by sizing the child's larynx with endotracheal tubes during laryngotracheobronchoscopic examination, and comparing this to normative tables of expected tube sizes in a child that age (see Figure 4.9.2).

9.6 How is the condition managed?

It is important to bear the diagnosis in mind. Where symptoms are suggestive, the diagnosis is made by formal laryngotracheobronchoscopy to examine the airway and assess the size and type of stenosis. In the context of failed extubation consideration should be given to optimizing any associated cardio-respiratory pathology, treating inflammatory changes with steroids and anti-reflux medication, and allowing a period of laryngeal rest. A cricoid split procedure may be required in more severe cases. In significant established stenoses other surgical options should be considered.

9.7 What are the main surgical options?

Tracheostomy may be required in the first instance. Most surgeons would regard 10kg as a minimum weight for a child to be able to have a good result from laryngeal augmentation surgery.

For grade I and II stenoses, limited endoscopic treatment may be attempted including cold steel/laser division of the stenosis +/– dilatation. In grade III and IV stenoses a more extensive procedure will be required. The options are augmentation grafting—either a single stage or two stage procedure with covering tracheostomy, and cricotracheal resection which is indicated for severe stenosis with a normal margin below the cords to allow anastomosis.

Stage	Grade I	Grade II	Grade III	Grade IV
From	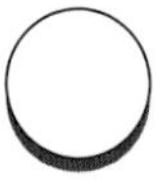 No obstruction	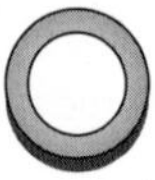 51% obstruction	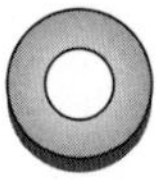 71% obstruction	No detectable lumen
To	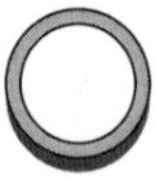 50% obstruction	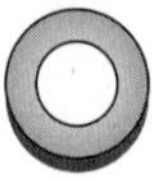 70% obstruction	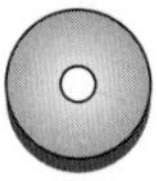 99% obstruction	

Figure 4.9.2 Adapted from *Pediatric ENT*, eds. John Graham, Glennis Scadding and Peter Bull, copyright 2008 with permission from Springer-Verlag.

Question 10

A 10-year-old child is brought to clinic with a midline neck swelling that moves upwards on swallowing and also moves on tongue protrusion.

10.1 What is the most likely diagnosis?

10.2 What is the differential diagnosis?

10.3 What is the embryological origin of thyroglossal duct cysts?

10.4 How would you manage an acutely infected thyroglossal duct cyst?

10.5 What investigations are indicated prior to surgery?

10.6 When is surgery indicated?

10.7 What are the important steps in the surgical approach?

10.8 How common are recurrences and how would you manage them?

Answers to Question 10

10.1 What is the most likely diagnosis?

A thyroglossal duct cyst.

10.2 What is the differential diagnosis?

- Thyroglossal duct cyst
- Lymph node/nodal abscess
- Dermoid cyst.

Theoretically, a thyroglossal duct cysts moves with tongue protrusion, but practically anything that is attached to the hyoid bone will move on tongue protrusion. An ultrasound scan is probably the most sensitive tool for discriminating between these pathologies.

10.3 What is the embryological origin of thyroglossal duct cysts?

The thyroid arises on 24th day of gestation as a diverticulum at the site of the foramen caecum between the anterior two-thirds and posterior one-third of the tongue. It descends to its final position at 7 weeks through the midline of the neck passing usually anterior, but closely related to the hyoid bone. The tract normally completely involutes prior to birth (7–10 weeks). Its persistence leads to the development of thyroglossal dust cysts.

10.4 How would you manage an acutely infected thyroglossal duct cyst?

Antibiotics (oral vs. IV depending on severity). If not settling consider aspiration. Avoid incision and drainage if possible to avoid a discharging sinus/fistula.

10.5 What investigations are indicated prior to surgery?

Ultrasound scan is useful both to confirm the presence of a normal thyroid gland and confirm that features of the swelling are consistent with the diagnosis.

10.6 When is surgery indicated?

In asymptomatic young children there is no indication for immediate surgery. Most ENT surgeons would advocate surgical excision at some point due to the high likelihood of developing infective complications and the very small risk of malignancy within the cyst (most commonly papillary thyroid cancer).

10.7 What are the important steps in the surgical approach?

Simple excision of the cyst results in 50%+ recurrence rates. Therefore, a more extensive procedure is indicated. This approach was described by Walter Sistrunk in 1920 (see Further reading) and involves removing the cyst and tract and mid portion of the hyoid and a wedge of tissue up into tongue base superior to the hyoid. There are some surgeons who prefer a wide excision approach including parts of the strap muscles to reduce the risk of leaving behind branches of the tract. The need for a drain is debated, although when post-operative bleeding does occur it can lead to rapid airway compromise.

10.8 How common are recurrences and how would you manage them?

Approximately 4% when a Sistrunk's-type procedure is performed. Management involves revision surgery with wider excision of the midline soft tissues and further hyoid resection.

Further reading

Sistrunk WE (1920). The surgical treatment of cysts of the thyroglossal tract. *Ann Surg* **71:** 121–2.

Question 11

11.1 Figure 4.11.1 is an intra-oral photograph. What does it show?

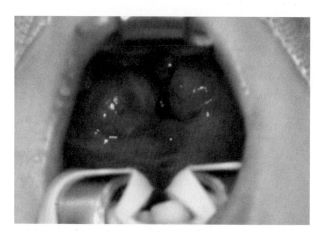

Figure 4.11.1

11.2 What symptoms is this child likely to present with?

11.3 How common are snoring and obstructive sleep apnoea (OSA) in children?

11.4 What is the difference between snoring and OSA?

11.5 Is OSA a common indication for tonsillectomy?

11.6 Do you know any risk factors for OSA?

11.7 What type of sleep studies can be used to assess the severity of sleep disordered breathing?

11.8 Which groups of children would you refer to a specialist centre for surgery?

Answers to Question 11

11.1 Figure 4.11.1 is an intra-oral photograph. What does it show?

A child with large obstructive tonsils.

11.2 What symptoms is this child likely to present with?

These are likely to include:
- *During the night*—snoring, struggling to breathe, witnessed apnoeas, unusual posture (neck extended), frequent waking, restlessness
- *During the day*—mouth breathing, stertor, poor concentration/behaviour
- *General*—poor feeding, especially for solids and poor growth.

11.3 How common are snoring and OSA in children?

Studies suggest snoring 10–20%, OSA 1–2%.

11.4 What is the difference between snoring and OSA?
- *Snoring*—the noise caused by turbulent airflow in upper respiratory tract (URT) without significant impairment of gas exchange and associated disrupted sleep
- *OSA*—disordered breathing due to prolonged partial/complete upper airway obstruction causing impaired ventilation and disrupted sleep
- *SBD*—(=sleep-related breathing disorders) encompasses the range of such disorders.

11.5 Is OSA a common indication for tonsillectomy?

It is becoming increasingly so. The commonest indication is recurrent tonsillitis, however in 2007–2008, a quarter of tonsillectomies done in children in the UK were for OSA.

11.6 Do you know any risk factors for OSA?
- Age 2–6 (maximal adenotonsillar hypertrophy)
- Down's syndrome
- Neuromuscular disorders
- Craniofacial abnormalities
- Obesity
- Achondroplasia
- Mucopolysaccharidoses.

11.7 What type of sleep studies can be used to assess the severity of sleep disordered breathing?

Overnight pulse oximetry

Can be a useful screening tool and has a high positive predictive value, however it is not able to reliably differentiate snoring from significant OSA with a negative predictive value of only around 50%. The gold standard investigation is polysomnography (involving at least oximetry, respiratory effort, airflow, ECG, and videotaping). This is not widely available therefore tends to be reserved for certain groups including those with diagnostic doubt, other significant co-morbidities, the very young (<2 years), and extremes of weight.

11.8 Which groups of children would you refer to a specialist centre for surgery?

- Age <2 years
- Weight <15kg
- Obesity
- *Comorbidity*—cerebral palsy, craniofacial abnormalities, mucopolysaccharidoses, significant cardio-respiratory disease
- Severe OSA on polysomnography (obstructive index >10, respiratory disturbance index >40, oxygen saturation nadir <80%).

Question 12

12.1 What does Figure 4.12.1 show?

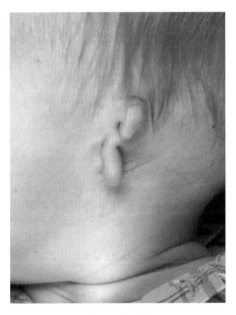

Figure 4.12.1

12.2 What would be your immediate concern?

12.3 When would you expect this to be picked up?

12.4 What type of hearing loss would you expect and how would you manage this?

12.5 Do you know of any grading systems for microtia?

12.6 Do you know of any associated conditions?

12.7 What other concerns are the parents likely to have and what are the options for managing this?

Answers to Question 12

12.1 What does Figure 4.12.1 show?

Baby with microtia.

12.2 What would be your immediate concern?

Likely association with significant hearing loss. If bilateral (15–30%) this has a much more serious impact on development and requires early intervention.

12.3 When would you expect this to be picked up?

At screening during the neonatal hearing screening programme. It is an indication for immediate referral for formal audiological assessment.

12.4 What type of hearing loss would you expect and how would you manage this?

Moderate to severe conductive loss. Embryologically, the external ear develops before the middle ear therefore significant microtia is almost always associated with middle ear abnormalities. Sensorineural function is usually normal as the development of the inner ear occurs at a separate embryological stage. In an infant with bilateral conductive loss a bone conduction hearing aid (usually on a soft band) should be provided as soon as possible with evidence that hearing outcomes are better in those aided before 6 months of age.

(The role of imaging to assess the middle and inner ear is controversial as surgical treatment for aural atresia is complex with limited success. Radiological grading of the anatomical abnormalities help to predict the likely outcome of surgery with only half of patients being potential candidates for repair. When surgery is contemplated the child needs to be a minimum of 5–6 years of age.)

12.5 Do you know of any grading systems for microtia?

Several different authors have described grading systems including Marx, Weerda and Aguilar, and Jahrsdoerfer. They are broadly similar:

- *Grade I*—abnormal shape, all anatomical subunits present
- *Grade II*—significant abnormality, some subunits present
- *Grade III*—severely deformed, usually with nubbin of cartilage superiorly and partial lobule only. Anotia also within this category (Weerda, Aguilar, and Jahrsdoerfer)
- *Grade IV*—anotia (Marx).

12.6 Do you know of any associated conditions?

- Microtia is associated with a syndrome in 5% of cases, but almost 30% have other associated abnormalities, but not with an eponymous syndrome
- Treacher Collins syndrome
- Goldenhar syndrome/hemifacial microsomia
- Trisomy 18 (Edwards syndrome)
- Maternal thalidomide exposure
- Foetal alcohol syndrome
- Maternal diabetes.

12.7 What other concerns are the parents likely to have and what are the options for managing this?

Parents are frequently concerned regarding the cosmetic appearance of the ears. It is routine practice to wait until the child is of an age where they can be actively involved in the decision regarding the need for treatment if at all. This is usually at around the age of 9–12 years. There are two main options—reconstruction, involving at least a two-stage procedure with cartilage harvest from the ribs, or a bone anchored prosthesis, which avoids prolonged surgery, but will need replacing at regular intervals as the child grows and with wear and tear.

Question 13

13.1 What is the NHSP?

13.2 What type of otoacoustic emission test is used in the NHSP in England and what are its limitations?

13.3 Do all children follow the same pathway?

13.4 What are risk factors for later onset deafness following the screening period?

13.5 Which groups of children are identified for further behavioural testing at 8 months even if they pass the initial screening test?

13.6 Is the NHSP cost effective?

Answers to Question 13

13.1 What is the NHSP?

This is a national screening programme carried out by trained hearing screeners/health visitors within 4 weeks of birth either in hospital or in the community. It was fully implemented in 2006 in England. Its aim is to identify children with a significant hearing loss defined as a permanent loss average >40dB in the better hearing ear.

13.2 What type of otoacoustic emission test is used in the NHSP in England and what are its limitations?

Transient evoked otoacoustic emissions. Parameters used are: click tone at 75–100pps, 80–88dB SPL, records 1–5kHz.

Limitations include:

- Can miss low frequency loss
- Response will be absent in OME
- Will miss losses further along auditory pathway than cochlea
- May miss losses which are progressive.

13.3 Do all children follow the same pathway?

Because of the increased risk of both overall and central auditory pathway hearing loss there is a different screening pathway for those who have spent >48h in SCBU/NICU.

- Well baby pathway (risk of hearing loss = 1:1000)—OAE alone with Automated ABR only if OAE response absent in one or both ears
- SCBU/NICU pathway (risk = 1:100)—both OAE and AABR for all (rationale being that neonates who have had hypoxic episodes have a higher incidence of retro cochlear auditory pathology).

13.4 What are risk factors for later onset deafness following the screening period?

The commonest is bacterial meningitis. Other causes include congenital CMV. temporal bone fracture, ototoxic drugs, hyperbilirubinaemia, and viral labyrinthitis, e.g. mumps and measles.

13.5 Which groups of children are identified for further behavioural testing at 8 months even if they pass the initial screening test?

- Syndromes associated with hearing loss/cleft palate/craniofacial abnormalities
- Missed screen or audiological follow-up.
- Family history in parents or siblings of permanent sensorineural hearing loss from childhood
- Mechanical ventilation >5 days, or extra-corporeal membrane oxygenation (ECMO)
- SCBU/NICU over 48h with no clear response OAE both ears despite clear response on AABR
- Severe jaundice or hyperbilirubinaemia
- Congenital infection due to one of the following: toxoplasmosis, rubella, cytomegalovirus
- Neurodegenerative or neurodevelopmental disorders
- Ototoxic drugs with monitored levels outside the therapeutic range.

13.6 Is the NHSP cost effective?

It replaced the health visitor distraction test (HVDT), which was not very sensitive. Relative cost calculations suggest that the new programme is cost effective:

HVDT = £20 000 per child fitted with hearing aid.
NHSP = £8–10 000 per child fitted with hearing aid.

Question 14

A teenage boy presents to your clinic with left-sided nasal obstruction and endoscopic examination is shown in Figure 4.14.1.

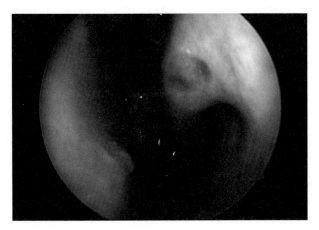

Figure 4.14.1

14.1 What is seen in Figure 4.14.1 and what is the differential diagnosis?

14.2 If the clinical diagnosis is of juvenile angiofibroma, what imaging investigations would you arrange and what are the typical appearances?

14.3 When and how would you expect this patient to present?

14.4 What histological features are typical?

14.5 Do you know any staging systems?

14.6 How would you manage the patient?

14.7 What surgical approaches can be used, and what guides your decision?

Answers to Question 14

14.1 What is seen in Figure 4.14.1 and what is the differential diagnosis?

This is a nasendoscopic photograph showing a fleshy mass occluding the left nasal cavity. The differential diagnosis in this age group includes juvenile angiofibroma, nasal polyp or inverted papilloma.

14.2 If the clinical diagnosis is of juvenile angiofibroma, what imaging investigations would you arrange and what are the typical appearances?

- *CT*—typical features include bowing of posterior wall of maxillary sinus (Hollman–Miller sign), erosion of floor of sphenoid, pterygoid plate. Mass is lobulated, enhancing and well demarcated
- *MRI*—useful in advanced disease to assess intracranial extension, relationship to dura and vessels. Appearance described as 'salt and pepper' with intense enhancement with gadolinium
- *Angiography*—not necessary for diagnosis, but useful for pre-operative embolization. Internal maxillary artery predominant vessel in 90–95%. Contralateral inferior meatal antrostomy (IMA) involved in more than 50%.

14.3 When and how would you expect this patient to present?

In an adolescent boy—median age 14 years. Commonest symptoms are nasal obstruction and recurrent severe epistaxis. In more advanced tumours—facial mass, proptosis, upper airway obstruction, cranial nerve palsies.

14.4 What histological features are typical?

No capsule. Irregular vascular component within a collagen rich stroma. The vascular channels lack smooth muscle and elastic fibres, which increases the severity of bleeding.

14.5 Do you know any staging systems?

There are many. One widely used is Radkowski (1996; see Further reading).

14.6 How would you manage the patient?

Main treatment is surgical. Radiotherapy has a place in widespread recurrences/inoperable disease, alone or in combination with surgical debulking which reduces radiation dose. Pre-operative embolization is carried out within 2–3 days of surgery.

14.7 What surgical approaches can be used, and what guides your decision?

Small tumours can be approached endoscopically. Larger/more extensive need midfacial degloving/lateral rhinotomy, or wider exposure with lateral skull base/infra-temporal approaches +/– neurosurgeon. Choice guided by the site and extent of tumour, and available expertise. Recurrence 20–50%.

Further reading

Radkowski D, McGill T, Healy GB, Ohlms L, Jones DT (1996). Angiofibroma. Changes in staging and treatment. *Arch Otolaryngol Head Neck Surg* **122**(2): 122–9.

Question 15

You are seeing a patient who is known to have laryngomalacia.

15.1 What is typically seen when a dynamic assessment is undertaken in these patients?

15.2 When and how does this condition usually present?

15.3 What are the key points in the history?

15.4 What are the other common causes of stridor in a baby and how do they differ in presenting features?

15.5 How would you manage the patient?

15.6 What is the surgical procedure described to treat the condition—briefly describe the key steps.

Answers to Question 15

15.1 What is typically seen when a dynamic assessment is undertaken in these patients?

Endoscopic examination typically shows a long curled (omega-shaped) epiglottis, bulky tall aryepiglottic folds, and evidence of collapse of these structures, which occurs during inspiration.

15.2 When and how does this condition usually present?

Laryngomalacia is the commonest cause of neonatal stridor. It typically presents at the age of 4–6 weeks, when inspiratory flow rates are high enough to generate the sound. The baby develops inspiratory stridor, which is characteristically high pitched and fluttering. It is most noticeable when the child is supine, and when they are active, e.g. during crying and feeding, and tends to increase as their activity levels increase in the first 9 months, thereafter gradually reducing, and usually resolving fully by about 2 years of age.

15.3 What are the key points in the history?

- What age did it start?
- Is the noise only present on inspiration?
- Is the child's voice (cry) normal?
- How well do they feed—do they tire, cough, choke?
- Have there been any episodes of apnoea or cyanosis?
- How is their weight gain? (Check the centile charts in the red book).

15.4 What are the other common causes of stridor in a baby and how do they differ in presenting features?

Examples are:
- *Vocal cord paralysis (uni-/bilateral)*—stridor may be inspiratory or biphasic, voice likely to be weak/breathy, tends to be present at birth
- *Subglottic haemangioma*—stridor biphasic, likely to progress more rapidly, may have a cutaneous haemangioma (50%), tends to present at 3–4 months
- *Subglottic stenosis (congenital/acquired)*—biphasic stridor. There is likely to be a history of (prolonged) intubation if stenosis is acquired
- *Tracheomalacia (primary/secondary)*—usually presents after 3 months of age, stridor—biphasic +/– wheeze, breathlessness, cough, apnoeic episodes.

15.5 How would you manage the patient?

Flexible nasendoscopy in the clinic is usually possible up to the age of 6 months. If this confirms the diagnosis and history is consistent with laryngomalacia, >90% of patients can be managed conservatively. Reflux laryngitis commonly co-exists, partly due to the increased intra-thoracic pressures generated by the partially obstructed airway; therefore, anti-reflux medication should be considered (gaviscon/ranitidine/omeprazole). In the remaining small percentage there are features of concern—including inconclusive history or examination, feeding difficulties/poor weight gain or a history of cyanotic/apnoeic episodes. These patients should be considered for surgical assessment and/or intervention depending on the degree of concern.

15.6 What is the surgical procedure described to treat the condition—briefly describe the key steps.

Supraglottoplasty/aryepiglottoplasty:

Key steps

- Start with full laryngotracheobronchosopy to assess the airway, confirm diagnosis and exclude any co-existing airway pathology
- Proceed to suspension microlarygoscopy. The baby may be intubated, or have a nasopharyngeal airway depending on surgeon/anaesthetist preference
- Aryepiglottic folds are divided. If needed excess mucosa is excised. If bulky arytenoids are present excising a small amount of cuneiform cartilage may also be considered.

Question 16

A child presents to your outpatient clinic because their mother is concerned about their drooling.

16.1 What points are important in the history?

16.2 What are the important examination features?

16.3 What are the non-surgical options for treating the problem?

16.4 What are the surgical options and what would determine your choice?

16.5 What are the risks of submandibular duct relocation?

Answers to Question 16

16.1 What points are important in the history?

- Age of the child (drooling is physiological up to age 2, and becomes a concern after age 5)
- *Comorbidities and general development*—drooling is much more common and problematic in children with associated neurological disabilities such as cerebral palsy
- Duration of the problem
- *Quantify it*—number of bib/clothes changes each day
- *Are there associated symptoms to suggest aspiration?*—chest infections/coughing or choking with feeding, use of NG or PEG feeding
- What measures have been tried to date?
- *Any regular medications*—anticonvulsants and nitrazepam increase saliva
- Is the child aware/distressed by it?

16.2 What are the important examination features?

- Head control
- Lip seal
- Tongue control
- Oral/perioral health
- Evidence of nasal obstruction (may exacerbate mouth open posture)
- Evidence of significant drooling.

16.3 What are the non-surgical options for treating the problem?

- Postural/oral awareness training if the child can benefit
- *Orthodontic*—malocclusion/palatal training devices
- *Anticholinergic medications*—hyoscine (usually patches), glycopyrrolate. Side effects especially dry mouth can be significant
- *Botulinum toxin*—injections with ultrasound guidance predominantly into submandibular glands. Needs repeating regularly. Useful and low morbidity to assess response before proceeding with more invasive surgery.

16.4 What are the surgical options and what would determine your choice?

- *Submandibular duct relocation*—not in those who aspirate. Otherwise tends to be first choice as no external scar and lower long-term morbidity
- *Submandibular gland excision*—better for those who aspirate. Risk of marginal mandibular nerve weakness
- *Parotid duct ligation*—usually only if other options have failed to give adequate improvement. Significant short-term swelling and discomfort.

16.5 What are the risks of submandibular duct relocation?

General

GA, bleeding, swelling, pain. Most common specific complication is ranula formation (5–10%). This is significantly reduced by the addition of sublingual gland excision to the procedure. However, this may increase morbidity related to pain and bleeding.

Question 17

17.1 What condition does this child shown in Figure 4.17.1 have and what features have led you to this conclusion?

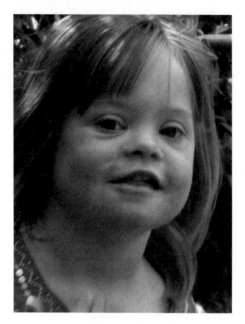

Figure 4.17.1

17.2 What is the genetic basis for this?

17.3 How common is it?

17.4 For what main reasons will the child present to an ENT surgeon?

17.5 How and why does management of otitis media with effusion differ from a child without Down's syndrome?

17.6 What extra precaution needs consideration if you perform an adenotonsillectomy for this child?

17.7 Would you expect their upper airway obstruction to fully resolve following adenotonsillectomy?

Answers to Question 17

17.1 What condition does this child shown in Figure 4.17.1 have and what features have led you to this conclusion?

Down's syndrome—Upslanting palpebral fissures, epicanthic folds, flat facial profile, small nose and ears, brachycephaly.

17.2 What is the genetic basis for this?

Trisomy 21 in the majority of cases, though can also be caused by translocations. There is a strong association with increasing maternal age (1 in 385 at age 35, 1 in 28 at age 45).

17.3 How common is it?

Approximately 1:1000 live births.

17.4 For what main reasons will the child present to an ENT surgeon?

- *Hearing loss*—may be sensorineural, conductive, or mixed
- Increased incidence of otitis media with effusion
- Rhinosinusitis
- Upper airway obstruction
- Subglottic stenosis (often mild and only recognized on intubation)
- Drooling.

Other features include:

- Developmental delay
- Hypotonia
- Congenital heart disease.

17.5 How and why does management of otitis media with effusion differ from a child without Down's syndrome?

OME is more common and tends to persist for longer. Anatomically, the external ear canals tend to be narrower. The resulting difficulty in inserting grommets, the fact that multiple sets of grommets may be needed and increased risk of otorrhoea following grommet insertion mean that a hearing aid should be considered as a preferable alternative to grommet insertion. (NICE Guidelines 2008—see Further reading).

17.6 What extra precaution needs consideration if you perform an adenotonsillectomy for this child?

There is a risk of atlantoaxial joint instability which is present 15% of the time and increases risk of subluxation. Therefore consider pre-operative C-spine x-rays, and limit neck extension during the procedure. Where there is a high index of suspicion of atlanto-axial joint instability, an MRI scan of the cervical spine should be considered as cervical spine plain radiology is not sufficiently sensitive.

17.7 Would you expect their upper airway obstruction to fully resolve following adenotonsillectomy?

Unlikely, as the obstruction tends to be multifactorial with contributions from macroglossia, hypotonia and narrow nasopharynx, as well as adenotonsillar obstruction.

Further reading

NICE (2008). *Surgical management of children with otitis media with effusion (OME)*, guideline CG60. Available at: http://guidance.nice.org.uk/CG60

Question 18

18.1 What are the clinical features of Treacher Collins syndrome?

18.2 What are the clinical features of Treacher Collins syndrome with regards to the ear?

18.3 What other syndromic causes of hearing loss do you know?

18.4 How would you subclassify causes of congenital hearing loss?

18.5 What environmental causes do you know?

18.6 What investigations would you arrange in a patient with unilateral sensorineural hearing loss?

18.7 Which healthcare and educational professionals would you expect to be involved in the care of a child with congenital deafness?

Answers to Question 18

18.1 What are the clinical features of Treacher Collins syndrome?

Maxillary hypoplasia, down-sloping palpebral fissures, telecanthus.

18.2 What are the clinical features of Treacher Collins syndrome with regards to the ear?

Microtia and aural atresia, ossicular abnormalities, increased incidence of OME, occasional cochlear abnormalities. Hearing loss is predominantly conductive.

18.3 What other syndromic causes of hearing loss do you know?

Autosomal dominant

- Waardenburg's syndrome
- Branchio-oto-renal syndrome
- Crouzon's syndrome
- Apert's syndrome
- Pierre Robin syndrome.

Autosomal recessive

- Pendred's syndrome
- Usher's syndrome
- Jervell–Lange-Nielsen syndrome
- Alport's syndrome.

18.4 How would you subclassify causes of congenital hearing loss?

Around 50% of cases are environmental and 50% genetic. Of genetic causes 30% are syndromic. Non-syndromic causes are predominantly autosomal recessive (80%), autosomal dominant account for 15%, x-linked 3%, and mitochondrial 2%. The commonest cause of autosomal recessive non-syndromal hearing loss is related to the Connexin 26 gene.

18.5 What environmental causes do you know?

- *Intrauterine infections*—toxoplasma, rubella, CMV, Herpes, HIV, syphilis
- *Toxins*—alcohol, tobacco, ototoxic medications
- *Birth history*—low birth weight, prolonged SCBU stay, hypoxia, hyperbilirubinaemia
- *Metabolic*—maternal diabetes, hypothyroidism.

18.6 What investigations would you arrange in a patient with unilateral sensorineural hearing loss?

This will depend on the mode of presentation and pointers in history and examination as to likely aetiology, but may include:

- Infection screen
- Urine dipstick
- Blood tests
- ECG
- Imaging-CT/MRI
- Renal USS
- Opthalmology review
- Genetic review.

18.7 Which healthcare and educational professionals would you expect to be involved in the care of a child with congenital deafness?

- Otolaryngologist
- Paediatrician
- Paediatric audiologist
- Speech therapist
- Teacher of the deaf.

Chapter 5

Operative surgery

Introduction

This section of the exam may be divided into three stations:
1. Temporal bone drilling (10min)
2. Nasal endoscopy (5min)
3. Prosections (5min).

Temporal bone drilling

You will be required to answer oral questions whilst performing this station. Do not stop your drilling to answer questions—you must continue to make progress in the dissection. Questions you might expect to arise include:

1. What is your inter-pupillary distance? *You will be expected to know this without hesitation.*
2. What speed is the drill supposed to be set to? Typically, a variable-speed drill is used, with a maximum speed of 90 000rev/min.
3. How do you choose your drill burr? You should choose the burr according to your anatomical location and requirements for speed of progress.
4. Which size of burr would you use to start a cortical mastoidectomy? A large cutting burr (e.g. 7mm) would be an appropriate starting size.
5. Where is the endolymphatic sac (ELS)? Donaldson's line is the superior limit of ELS (see Figures 5.1 and 5.2).
6. What are the indications for a cortical mastoidectomy?
- *Access CAT:*
  - Ossiculoplasty
  - Cochlear implant
  - Endolymphatic sac surgery

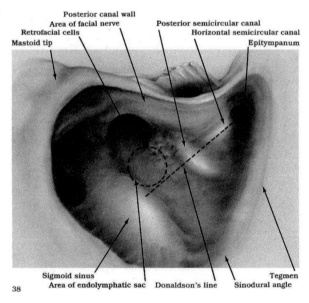

38

Figure 5.1. Right mastoid dissection. Image courtesy of the House Research Institute.

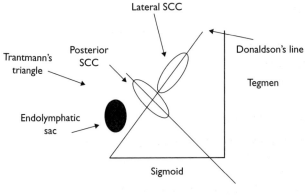

Figure 5.2

- ◆ Facial nerve decompression
- ◆ IAM access
- In combination with a myringoplasty
- Acute mastoiditis.
7. What are the landmarks of the facial nerve?
- Digastric ridge
- Inferior to the lateral SCC
- Stylomastoid foramen/tympanomastoid suture
- Superior to stapes footplate
- Above cochleariform process—reliable as unlikely to be eroded by disease.
8. What are the indications for a posterior tympanotomy?
- CAT
- Cochlear implant
- Middle ear implant
- Ossiculoplasty.
9. What are the landmarks for a posterior tympanotomy
- Buttress over SPI
- Chorda tympani
- Incus
- 2nd genu of facial nerve
- Tympanic membrane.
10. What would you do if you caused a CSF leak?
- Insert temporalis fascia between the dura and the bone or fat/muscle over bone, and Tisseel
- Insert bone pâté.
11. What would you do with a fistula of the lateral SCC during cholesteatoma surgery?
- Expect a fistula in everyone—whether there is radiological evidence or not
- Do the bony work first. Then:
  - ◆ if able to remove all matrix, do so, cover with fascia, and plan a second look *or*
  - ◆ if unable to remove the matrix, convert to MR mastoidectomy and matrix will form part of squamous lining of cavity.

12. What would you do if you caused a bleed from the sigmoid sinus?
- If small bony defect, bone wax
- If larger defect, rotate a muscle flap into the defect or fascia then free muscle or fat with Tisseel over area.
13. In the recovery room following mastoid surgery, your patient has a facial nerve palsy. What are you going to do?
- Wait for the local anaesthetic to wear off
- If you are **sure** the nerve was intact during surgery, remove packing
- If you are not sure the nerve was intact, re-explore the ear with a colleague assisting.
14. What are the landmarks of the mastoid antrum?
- 1.5cm deep to McEwan's triangle in an adult
- Cribriform area of bone due to perforating vessels (provide pathway of spread of infection to subperiosteal space in mastoiditis).
15. What is Koerner's septum? The petrosquamous suture.

Rigid nasal endoscopy

Be familiar with how to set up the endoscope, including focus and white balance.
- *Three passes:*
  - *Floor of nose into nasopharynx*—pay attention to inferior meatus; inspect post-nasal space, including Eustachian tube orifices and fossa of Rosenmüller
  - *Under middle turbinate*—examine middle meatus; pass endoscope medial to middle turbinate to examine spheno-ethmoidal recess and sphenoid ostium
  - If possible, examine olfactory cleft.
- *Questions relating to FESS:*
  - How to perform certain steps
  - *Complications*—e.g. CSF leak.

Prosections

Skull base and its foramina
- *Mandible*—landmarks, muscle insertions, embryology
- *Hyoid*—landmarks, muscle insertions, embryology
- *Neck landmarks in prosection:*
  - Point out triangles of the neck
  - Point out demarcations of level I/IIa/IIb/III/IV/V
- *Questions relating to anatomy of certain surgical procedures:*
  - Neck dissections
  - Submandibular gland excision.

Chapter 6

Clinical stations

Introduction

This section of the examination is divided into two 20-min sections. In each section, you can expect to see two patients, each for 10min.

In the clinical examination part of Fellow of the Royal College of Surgeons (FRCS), you will encounter patients with clinical conditions. You will be required to examine them and present your findings to the examiners. Questioning may then lead on to investigations and management of the conditions you see.

There are a few basic, but very key points to bear in mind for this part of the examination:

1 Present yourself as you would for your normal clinical practice: look smart. The rule of 'bare below the elbows' applies in this examination: if you choose to wear a tie, this should either be tucked into your shirt, or held in place with a tie clip.
2 Under no circumstances must you hurt the patient. This is viewed very dimly indeed by the examiners.
3 Use the alcohol hand gel that will be provided at all the stations. Alternatively, bring your own to attach to your belt.
4 Listen carefully to what the examiner says. If (s)he says, 'Examine this patient's thyroid gland', then examine the neck. If (s)he says, 'Examine this patient's thyroid status', then you should start with a general physical examination, including pulse, skin, etc.
5 Patients will generally have chronic conditions that do not render them acutely unwell. It is likely, therefore, that you will encounter conditions such as stable neck lumps (e.g. parotid, thyroid), children with syndromes, patients with ear implants (BAHA, cochlear implants).

This chapter proposes a suggested sequence for examination of different systems. Be methodical and systematic in your examination—do not attempt to take short cuts.

The examiner may try to rush you through different aspects of the examination. In part, this is to ensure that you have time to gain points in the exam. You must remember to offer to complete the examination ('... and, of course, I would like to perform tuning fork testing and clinical tests of hearing...'). Do not allow yourself to be flustered by the examiner—even if you do not have time to perform a full examination, you must remember to offer to complete the components you have not yet done.

Ear examination

- Take off glasses
- Remove hearing aid(s)
- *Inspect for:*
  - ◆ Post-auricular scar
  - ◆ Pits
  - ◆ Endaural scar
- *Otoscopy:*
  - ◆ Canal
  - ◆ TM/attic/cavity
  - ◆ Ossicles
- *Pneumatic otoscopy*
- *Tuning forks:*
  - ◆ Weber
  - ◆ Rinne

- Clinical tests of hearing (see below)
- Full ENT examination including nose, PNS
- Facial nerve.
- Neck.

In addition, offer to perform:

- Pure tone audiometry, tympanometry
- Speech audiometry
- Objective tests
- *Stenger*—a clinical test designed to determine malingering patients who are feigning a unilateral hearing loss. It relies on the principle that, when both ears are presented with a tone of identical pitch, but differing intensities, the sound will only be perceived as coming from the louder side. By the same token, two tones of the same intensity will appear to originate from the midline. Stand behind the patient with two tuning forks of the same pitch:
  - First, strike a tuning fork and hold it 15cm from the 'good' ear. The patient will confirm that they can hear the tone
  - Then hold a ringing tuning fork 5cm from the 'bad' ear. The patient will deny being able to hear it
  - Finally, out of sight of the patient, simultaneously hold one ringing tuning fork 15cm from the 'good' ear and another 5cm from the 'bad' ear. If the patient is genuinely deaf in the 'bad' ear, they will hear the sound in the better ear. If they are feigning hearing loss, they will deny hearing either sound.

Clinical tests of hearing

Candidates are frequently asked to perform these tests. You should practice with colleagues so that you become familiar with how to look slick at undertaking these tests.

- Explain procedure to patient
- Stand behind patient—shield your mouth
- *Adults*—use number-letter-number, e.g. 4-A-8
- *Children*—use two syllable words, e.g. cowboy; teacup
- Test better ear first
- *Mask non-test ear with tragal rubbing*—~50dB attenuation
- The threshold for normal hearing is said to be when the patient correctly identifies >50% of words
- Start with a whisper at arm's length—i.e. about 34dB (see Table 6.1).
- In practice, if the patient can hear a whispered voice at arm's length, the hearing is likely to be virtually normal.

Distance	Example	Voice	dB
12ft = 4m	Across a room	Whisper	<20dB
2ft = 60cm	Arm's length	Whisper	<25dB
6in = 15cm		Whisper	34dB
2ft = 60cm	Arm's length	Conversational	48dB
6in = 15cm		Conversational	56dB
6in = 15cm		Loud voice	75dB

Table 6.1 Rough guide to sound intensities in clinical tests of hearing

Neck examination

- *Inspection*—remember to inspect the patient and the surrounding room as you walk in, e.g. there may be a glass of water or an electrolarynx:
  - ◆ Offer to expose down to nipples (but to shoulders will usually suffice)
  - ◆ Take off HME if the patient has a stoma.
  - ◆ Abdomen for PEG
  - ◆ Scars on the arm suggesting a free flap, or on the chest for a pec major or delto-pectoral flap
  - ◆ *Sip water*—thyroid/thyroglossal duct cyst
  - ◆ *Stick tongue out*—thyroglossal duct cyst
- *Palpation*—submental (SM), parotid, post-auricular, levels II, III, IV, anterior compartment, level IV, V, occiput
- *Mouth:*
  - ◆ Remove dentures
  - ◆ Using two tongue depressors, thoroughly examine the whole oral cavity, including buccal sulci, roof of mouth, floor of mouth, and retromolar trigone
- Perform full ENT examination including ears, nose, scalp
- Flexible nasendoscopy
- Facial nerve/other CNs
- Auscultate neck.

A huge variety of clinical conditions can be seen in the head & neck section of the exam. A few common conditions include:

- Parotid mass (remembering to examine the facial nerve and the parotid duct orifice)
- Laryngectomy
- Pectoralis major flap
- *Free flap*—free radial forearm, fibular flap, etc.
- *Neck incision*—know the names of the common neck incisions, and what they are used for
- Facelift incision/parotidectomy scar
- *Jaw split incision (lip split mandibulotomy)*—for access to floor of mouth, oral cavity, and oropharynx.

Thyroid examination

- Inspect; swallow
- *Palpate:*
  - ◆ Swallow
  - ◆ lymph node (LN) areas
- *Eyes:*
  - ◆ Exophthalmos
  - ◆ Lid lag
- *Hands*—tremor, skin quality
- Pulse
- *Reflexes*—slow relaxing in hypothyroidism
- Proximal muscle wasting in hypo- and hyperthyroidism.

Nose examination

- *Inspect:*
  - Remove spectacles
  - Frontal, lateral, basal, and superior views
  - Skin thickness
  - Alignment, width, tip, base, profile, projection, rotation (chin)
  - Facial proportions
- Fogging
- Push up nasal tip for columella dislocation
- Thudichum
- Rigid/flexible endoscopy
- Full ENT examination, including oral cavity, neck, ears, and facial sensation
- *Tests:*
  - University of Pennsylvania Smell Identification Test (UPSIT)
  - Acoustic rhinometry
  - Rhinomanometry
  - Peak expiratory nasal flow.

Clinical entities you may expect to see:

- *Wegener's granulomatosis*—septal perforation; saddle deformity; crusting
- Other causes of septal perforation
- Lupus pernio
- *Lateral rhinotomy scar*—this may lead on to a discussion about nasal tumours, inverted papilloma, etc.
- Congenital deformities
- Cleft
- *Previous surgery*—e.g. open rhinoplasty, Lynch–Howarth incision.

Syndromic child

- NG/PEG
- Mouth-breathing
- Tracheostomy/scar
- *Facies:*
  - Midface
  - Occiput
  - Eye spacing
  - Coloboma
- *Ears:*
  - Low-set
  - Lop
  - Microtia
  - Scars
  - BAHA/HA
- *Mouth/jaw:*
  - Macroglossia
  - Micrognathia
- Facial nerve.

Syndromes to expect
- Down's
- Apert's
- Crouzon's
- Pierre-Robin
- Treacher–Collins.

Chapter 7

Communication skills

Introduction

The communication part of the examination is sometimes seen as a daunting component of the exam. However, in many ways, it is an opportunity to relax, and to try and replicate what you do in the clinic every week.

There is usually an actor who will have been given a scenario in advance. You will also be given some background information. However, be aware that the actor may have different information from you.

The scenarios will try to imitate situations you would be expected to encounter in the outpatient setting. The examiners will be looking at your ability to assimilate the information you have been given and how you communicate with the patient.

During the exam be prepared for the examiners to advance the situation; this often reflects that things are going well. An example of this would be a scenario involving a consultation, then the consent process, and then perhaps the follow-up consultation.

The scenario, as well as judging your communication skills, will also often have a knowledge component. An example of this would be when consenting to describe the potential complications, recognizing the risk of these, and addressing any concerns the patient may have. The examiners will be looking for you to use appropriate language.

This chapter gives some scenarios that mirror the type that are asked. It is impossible to describe what to say word by word as this will vary depend on your individual approach to the situation and will also be a dynamic situation. However, certain points that may need to be explored in each scenario are listed. Ideally, practising with a colleague or friend is the ideal way to prepare for this part of the exam.

Before you go in:

- Try to remember you are in the clinic and if in doubt, do what you would do there
- Decide if you are going to shake hands
- Remember try not to assume that the actor has the same information you do—much as in a normal clinic setting.

When you go in/they come in:

- Introduce yourself
- Try to smile and relax.

The scenarios in this chapter illustrate the types of situations that have been used in the past.

Scenarios

Scenario 1

You are in clinic with the results of a sleep study conducted on a gentleman the previous month by your registrar. He has a body mass index (BMI) of 45 and his apnoea score is 75. He is a heavy goods vehicle driver.

Points:

- Discuss the diagnosis of obstructive sleep apnoea (OSA)
- The effects of OSA and tiredness
- Likely treatment options
- *Implications for driving*—in this scenario he may be unwilling to inform the DVLA and so understanding your responsibilities is important.

The General Medical Council (GMC) have produced guidelines regarding this. The guidelines in Box 7.1 are taken from the guidelines at the time of writing (GMC, 2009).

Box 7.1 GMC Guidelines on Confidentiality: reporting concerns about patients to the DVLA or the DVA, GMC 2009

4. The driver is legally responsible for informing the DVLA or DVA about such a condition or treatment. However, if a patient has such a condition, you should explain to the patient that:

   - The condition may affect their ability to drive (if the patient is incapable of understanding this advice, for example, because of dementia, you should inform the DVLA or DVA immediately)
   - They have a legal duty to inform the DVLA or DVA about the condition.

5. If a patient refuses to accept the diagnosis or the effect of the condition on their ability to drive, you can suggest that they seek a second opinion, and help arrange for them to do so. You should advise the patient not to drive in the meantime.

6. If a patient continues to drive when they may not be fit to do so, you should make every reasonable effort to persuade them to stop. As long as the patient agrees, you may discuss your concerns with their relatives, friends, or carers.

7. If you do not manage to persuade the patient to stop driving or you discover that they are continuing to drive against your advice, you should contact the DVLA or DVA immediately, and disclose any relevant medical information, in confidence, to the medical adviser.

8. Before contacting the DVLA or DVA you should try to inform the patient of your decision to disclose personal information. You should then also inform the patient in writing once you have done so.

Reproduced with permission from the GMC's *'Guidelines on Confidentiality: reporting concerns about patients to the DVLA or the DVA'*, Copyright GMC 2009.

Box 7.2 GMC Guidelines 0–18 years: guidance for all doctors, GMC 2007

31. Parents cannot override the competent consent of a young person to treatment that you consider is in their best interests. However, you can rely on parental consent when a child lacks the capacity to consent. In Scotland, parents cannot authorize treatment a competent young person has refused. In England, Wales, and Northern Ireland, the law on parents overriding young people's competent refusal is complex. You should seek legal advice if you think treatment is in the best interests of a competent young person who refuses.

(Continued)

> **Box 7.2 (Continued)**
>
> 32. You must carefully weigh up the harm to the rights of children and young people of overriding their refusal against the benefits of treatment, so that decisions can be taken in their best interests. In these circumstances, you should consider involving other members of the multi-disciplinary team, an independent advocate, or a named or designated doctor for child protection. Legal advice may be helpful in deciding whether you should apply to the court to resolve disputes about best interests that cannot be resolved informally.
>
> 33. You should also consider involving these same colleagues before seeking legal advice if parents refuse treatment that is clearly in the best interests of a child or young person who lacks capacity, or if both a young person with capacity and their parents refuse such treatment
>
> Reproduced with permission from the GMC's '*Guidelines 0–18 years: guidance for all doctors*' Copyright GMC 2007.

Scenario 2

A 7-year-old girl is admitted via A&E with acute stridor. A diagnosis of acute epiglottitis has been made. You feel that she requires intubation for her airway. However, her father is concerned and does not want her to have a general anaesthetic while her mother is not here. Her mother is currently flying back from France.

Points:

- In this situation it is important to explain the seriousness of the situation to the father
- You should also explain the need for early intervention and the consequences of delay
- You may want to offer to involve another consultant as a second opinion
- Your priority is to your patient, the child, and their best interests (see Box 7.2).

Scenario 3

A patient presents to clinic as a 2-week wait referral with stridor. On nasendoscopy he has a T4 transglottic tumour with a 'pinhole' airway. Your opinion is that the patient needs to go to theatre as an emergency. Consent the patient for theatre.

In this instance, the patient does not want to have a tracheostomy.

Points:

- It is important to try and ascertain what the patient understands about there condition
- Stress that this would only be done if it was a life-threatening situation
- Involve another professional such as the anaesthetist.

Scenario 4

A 12-year-old patient is admitted to A&E with a post-tonsillectomy bleed. He has a Hb of 6g/dl and is actively bleeding. He is accompanied by his father and both are Jehovah's witnesses. Consent the patient for theatre.

In this situation the father and son do not want a blood transfusion.

Points:

- It is important to be respectful of their religious views
- Try to involve the patient and parent in all decisions
- As stated in the GMC guidance you can provide emergency treatment without consent to save the life of, or prevent serious deterioration in the health of a child or young person.

The GMC has issued guidance on this (see Box 7.3).

Scenario 5

A 45-year-old man comes to clinic with left otosclerosis. He wants to discuss the options of stapedectomy surgery. He is otherwise fit and well, and works as a self-employed roofer. Discuss the operation and risks.

Points:

- You should be able to describe the operation
- You should discuss the risks and the incidence of them
- You should discuss the risk of vertigo post-operatively and how this may affect his ability to work
- Alternatives to surgery should be discussed.

Scenario 6

A 50-year-old lady comes to clinic with her husband. She underwent a panendoscopy and biopsy last week of a T4 post-criciod tumour. She is a non-smoker. Histology confirms this is a squamous cell carcinoma. She has had an MRI of her neck and chest CT is reported as normal (staging is T4 N0 M0). She has been discussed at the MDT earlier and the consensus opinion was that she should be offered a laryngo-pharyngo/oesophagectomy. Discuss the diagnosis and implications of treatment with her.

Points:

- This involves breaking bad news, try to ascertain what she has been told what she understands about treatment
- Be sensitive to her questions
- Discuss the implications of surgery with her and, in particular, the effects on speech and swallowing
- Be prepared to discuss alternative options, survival, and the cause of her cancer
- Offer her some written information (have a look what information is given out in your MDT and quote that)
- It may be appropriate to offer to meet her again to go over the diagnosis and treatment plan
- The clinical nurse specialist should be involved and they may see her separately
- It may be appropriate to arrange a meeting with a patient who has undergone a similar procedure.

Scenario 7

You are in clinic with an 18-year-old boy and his parents. He has unaidable hearing loss following a peri-natal infection. He currently signs and is otherwise well. He and his parents wish to discuss the options of a cochlear implant.

Points:

- It is important to try and understand why he is now considering a cochlear implant
- What are his expectations given that he is pre-lingually deaf?

Scenario 8

A 10-year-old boy presents with a left cholesteotoma. Discuss the options of surgery, including the complications. In this scenario the actor playing the parent is unwilling to consider surgery.

Points:

- Explain the nature and behaviour of a cholesteotoma
- Explain what surgery would involve
- Explain the risks of surgery
- If the parents refuse surgery and given that this is not a life-threatening situation, then referring the patient for a second opinion may be the best option (see Box 7.2).

Scenario 9

A 45-year-old man has asked to see you again. He is accompanied by his partner. He has never smoked and drinks socially. Last week he was diagnosed with a T2 N0 M0 left tonsil tumour. He is aware of the diagnosis and treatment is planned. Last week when he was seen he was told that this was a p16 positive squamous cell carcinoma. He has since done some research on the internet and is concerned that his tumour has occurred because of a sexually-transmitted disease. He also wants to know if his son should be vaccinated.

Points:

- Establish what information he has found
- Be sensitive that he is with his wife and that this information may be of concern to both of them
- Describe the relationship of p16 immunohistochemistry and HPV infection
- Describe the association of HPV and oropharyngeal cancer
- Be aware of the incidence of HPV in the general population
- Discuss current national vaccination policy for HPV.

Scenario 10

A patient for a total laryngectomy is listed for surgery. At 08.30 hours you are informed by the bed manager that there is no bed today and no prospect of one. The patient was cancelled last week for the same problem. Explain to the patient and their relatives that their operation has to be cancelled.

Points:

- Explain the situation
- Be sensitive to the frustrations of the patient and family
- Be clear on what you plan to do to ensure a list is arranged
- Be careful not to make promises that you cannot guarantee, such as this will be done next week
- Ensure you know your local hospital's policy for complaints.

Scenario 11

You are seeing a 35-year-old male patient with ill-defined headaches. The patient has previously seen a neurologist who diagnosed tension headaches. The patient wants an MRI scan. In this situation the patient has a relative who died of a brain tumour.

Points:

- It is important to take a thorough history
- Understanding what the patient is concerned about is important
- In this situation, a tumour is very unlikely and MRI is probably not appropriate.

Scenario 12

A patient comes to see you having had a septoplasty performed 3 months previously by your registrar. The patient still has nasal obstruction and on examination has a large septal perforation. The operation note is missing from the notes and the patient has waited 3h to see you, while the note was looked for.

Points:

- It is important to recognize the frustrations the patient may have with both the long wait and the fact that their obstruction is still present
- You need to explain the findings of the perforation and that this is a recognized complication
- Acknowledge that the operation note is not present and explain what you will do
- Discuss further treatment options
- It may be necessary to offer a second opinion.

Scenario 13

A 40-year-old patient underwent resection of a malignant parotid tumour 12 months ago. A CXR has revealed widespread metastatic disease. He is married and father to two small children. He is the main income generator for the family. Discuss the findings with him and his wife.

Points:

- This involves breaking bad news
- Try to ascertain what he has been told, if anything
- Be sensitive to questions
- Discuss the findings of chest metastasis
- Be prepared to discuss palliative care and survival
- It may be appropriate to offer to meet her again to go over the diagnosis
- The clinical nurse specialist should be involved and they may see her separately.

Scenario 14

You are seeing a 3-year-old boy who has had two episodes of tonsillitis in the last year. He is otherwise fit and well and does not snore. His sister had her tonsils removed at the age of 8 after many years of repeated tonsillitis. His mother is insistent that she wants to have his tonsils removed.

Points:

- Clarify what they mean by tonsillitis and the number of episodes
- Understand the local guidelines for tonsillectomy
- Explain the risks of surgery
- You may need to offer a second opinion.

Scenario 15

You are seeing a 1-year-old child who is not reaching his milestones. He is with his mother. He suffered from viral meningitis aged 3 months. His parents are divorced and his mother is a solicitor. Audiometry shows a bilateral severe sensorineural hearing loss. Discuss the findings.

Points:

- Explain the findings of the hearing test
- Discuss the need for hearing aids (and also possibly cochlear implantation)
- Involve support services.

Scenario 16

A 56-year-old man presents with bilateral (non-pulsatile) tinnitus. He has a normal audiogram. He is very distressed by the tinnitus and has been told that there is no cure.

Points:

- Ascertain what problems it is causing him
- Explain the theories of tinnitus

> **Box 7.4 GMC Guidelines 0–18 years: guidance for all doctors, GMC 2007**
>
> 30. Respect for young people's views is important in making decisions about their care. If they refuse treatment, particularly treatment that could save their life or prevent serious deterioration in their health, this presents a challenge that you need to consider carefully.
>
> 31. Parents cannot override the competent consent of a young person to treatment that you consider is in their best interests. But you can rely on parental consent when a child lacks the capacity to consent. In Scotland parents cannot authorize treatment a competent young person has refused. In England, Wales and Northern Ireland, the law on parents overriding young people's competent refusal is complex. You should seek legal advice if you think treatment is in the best interests of a competent young person who refuses.
>
> Reproduced with permission from the GMC's 'Guidelines 0–18 years: guidance for all doctors' Copyright GMC 2007.

- Discuss natural the history of tinnitus
- Discuss treatment strategies
- Consider tinnitus counselling
- Written information may help, and he may wish to join a support group.

Scenario 17

A 14-year-old boy is listed for a tonsillectomy for recurrent tonsillitis. He is in the anaesthetic room with his mother. He now decides that he does not want surgery. His mother is cross because she wants him to have it as he is missing lots of school. The actor plays the role of the mother.

Points:

- Discuss with the boy and the mother the surgical procedure
- Try to understand what the concerns are
- It may be appropriate to send the boy back to the ward and re-send later.

The GMC (0–18 years: guidance for all doctors) (see Boxes 7.3 and 7.4) is clear that you can provide medical treatment to a child or young person with their consent if they are competent to give it.

Scenario 18

A 90-year-old man presents to A&E with stridor. He is visiting his family from another city. Clinically, he has an obstructing laryngeal tumour. He needs a tracheostomy as an emergency. Discuss this with him.

Points:

- Important to explain the findings in A&E
- Be prepared to have an answer regarding the cause of the obstruction
- Do not second guess the pathology, but you may be asked if it is cancer
- Explain what a tracheostomy is for and how he will function with it
- Be prepared to discuss what will happen after the tracheostomy—await pathology and imaging.

Further reading

GMC (2009). *Guidelines on Confidentiality: reporting concerns about patients to the DVLA or the DVA.* London: GMC.

Items should be returned on or before the last date shown below. Items not already requested by other borrowers may be renewed in person, in writing or by telephone. To renew, please quote the number on the barcode label. To renew online a PIN is required. This can be requested at your local library.
Renew online @ **www.dublincitypubliclibraries.ie**
Fines charged for overdue items will include postage incurred in recovery. Damage to or loss of items will be charged to the borrower. *223.2047*

**Leabharlanna Poiblí Chathair Bhaile Átha Cliath
Dublin City Public Libraries**

Date Due	Date Due	Date Due

Folio 21r of the *Cathach* showing initial *M* and beginning of Psalm 56.

The *Cathach* of Colum Cille

An introduction

by

Michael Herity

and

Aidan Breen

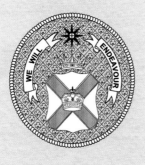

Royal Irish Academy

2002

First published in 2002
by the Royal Irish Academy
19 Dawson Street
Dublin 2
Ireland
www.ria.ie

British Library Cataloguing-in-Publication Data
A catalogue record for this publication is available from the
British Library.
ISBN 1-874045-92-5 (with CD-ROM)
1-874045-97-6 (without CD-ROM)

Design and layout by Martello Media Ltd, Dublin
Printed in Ireland by ColourBooks Ltd, Dublin

Contents

vi

Acknowledgements

The Royal Irish Academy wishes to acknowledge a substantial anonymous donation without which the publication of the *Cathach* CD-ROM and booklet would not have been possible.

The Academy's Dictionary of Medieval Latin from Celtic Sources project, whose staff (especially Anthony Harvey, Christopher Sweeney and Angela Malthouse) prepared the digital edition of H.J. Lawlor's transcription of the *Cathach* manuscript for the CD-ROM, made a significant contribution to the project.

The assistance of the Academy's library staff and the advice of the Librarian, Siobhán O'Rafferty, are gratefully acknowledged. Thanks are also due to David Cooper of Digital Lightforms Ltd, Oxfordshire, for assistance with the project.

Mrs Harriet Sheehy kindly gave permission for digital reproduction of extracts from Maurice Sheehy's work on the Springmount Bog wax tablets.

The authors of the booklet wish to thank F.J. Byrne, Anthony Cains, Martin McNamara and Timothy O'Neill for their contributions towards the research on the manuscript. The contribution of Marcus Redmond, who acted as research assistant to Professor Michael Herity, is also gratefully acknowledged.

Permission to reproduce illustrations in which copyright is held by persons or institutions other than the Royal Irish Academy is gratefully acknowledged.

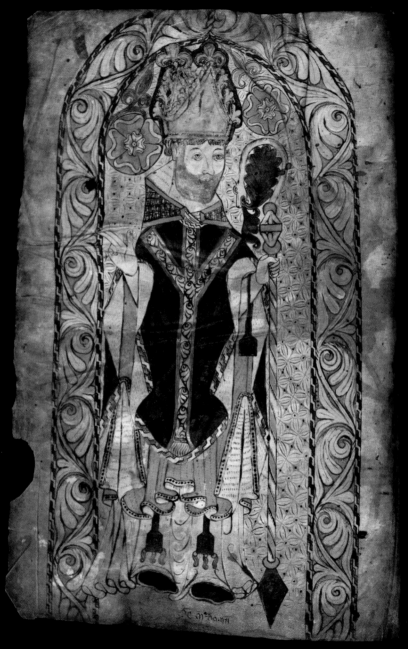

Image of Colum Cille, fol. iii v of Bodleian Library MS Rawl. B. 514 (Maghnus Ó Domhnaill's sixteenth-century Life of Colum Cille). (© Bodleian Library, University of Oxford, 2002)

Introduction

The *Cathach* is a manuscript of the Psalms in a relatively pure Gallican version of St Jerome's Latin Vulgate. The earliest extant Irish illuminated manuscript, it has been dated to *c.* AD 600 and is traditionally regarded as written by Colum Cille (Alexander 1978, 28–9). With its *cumhdach* or metal shrine, it was placed in in the care of the Royal Irish Academy in 1843 by the O'Donel family of Newport, County Mayo, who brought it back to Ireland, probably from Flanders (modern Belgium), in the early nineteenth century. To our knowledge, it is the only surviving Irish psalter for which a metal book-shrine was made.[1]

Colum Cille (521–97) was born at Gartan, County Donegal, according to his twelfth-century Irish Life (Herbert 1988, 275 n. 173). His father was Fedelmith, grandson of Conall, the eponymous ancestor of the kings of Tír Conaill; his mother was Eithne, who was of royal Leinster ancestry according to tenth-century sources (Ó Riain 1985, 76). He was fostered by a priest called Cruithnechán, studied as a deacon under Gemmán the Master in Leinster, later with Bishop Finnian, probably Finnian of Mag Bile (Moville, County Down), who died in 579, and, according to his Irish Life, with Mo Bí at Glasnevin.[2] Maghnus Ó Domhnaill, Lord of Tír Conaill from 1537 to 1555, related that Colum Cille spent some time as a hermit at Glend Colaim Cilli (Gleann Choluim Cille) in south-west County Donegal, where there are typical remains of an appropriately early date at the west end of the valley (Herity 1989, 95–106, 119–23). Colum Cille founded the monasteries of Durrow, Kilmore—the latter correctly identified by Reeves (1857, 173–4) as Kilmore, County Cavan—and Iona (Í Coluim Chille) in Scotland. Derry (Herbert 1988, 31) was founded or refounded, possibly in Colum Cille's lifetime, by his cousin Fiachra mac Ciaráin, who died in 620. The Columban federation later included Lambay (founded in 635), Drumcliff, Swords, Moone

---

[1] The scope of this booklet, which focuses on the *Cathach* manuscript, does not allow for a full discussion of its *cumhdach*, or shrine. A full description by E.C.R. Armstrong (1916), however, forms Appendix I of H.J. Lawlor's (1916) extensive essay on the *Cathach*.

[2] A list of Irish placenames mentioned in this booklet, with the counties in which they are located, can be found in Appendix 1.

and many other churches in Ireland as well as those of the *paruchia* in Scotland and Northumbria. After the Viking devastation of Iona, a *nova civitas* was founded at Kells in 807. The Columban church in Scotland likewise received a new metropolis at Dunkeld. By the twelfth century Derry had replaced Kells as the head of the *paruchia* (Herbert 1988, 113–23). The Annals of Ulster (AU), based on an early Iona chronicle and later continued at Armagh, were being redacted at Derry towards the end of the twelfth century or possibly earlier. From the tenth century until the beginning of the thirteenth century attempts were made from time to time to revive the unity of the Scottish and Irish federation under Iona.

A legend first attested in the late Middle Ages states that on a visit to St Finnian of Druim Fhinn (place unidentified), perhaps Bishop Finnian of Moville, who is credited with bringing the 'complete Gospels in a single volume' (probably the Vulgate) to Ireland, Colum Cille discovered a book and secretly made a copy of it. Maghnus Ó Domhnaill identified this copy with the *Cathach*. Finnian claimed that the copy rightfully belonged to him and referred the matter to Diarmait mac Cerbaill, King of Tara. The king's judgment, recorded by Ó Domhnaill (O'Kelleher and Schoepperle 1918, §168), has been cited as one of the oldest references to the idea of copyright (Fig. 1):

> 'le gach boin a boinin' .i. a laogh ⁊ 'le gach
> lebhur a leabrán'
> (This may be translated as 'To every cow her
> calf, so to every book its copy'.)

According to the legend, this led to the battle of Cúl Drebene, probably fought at modern Cooldrumman, 3km north of Drumcliff, opposite Ben Bulben in County Sligo, where an alliance of northern rulers that included Colum Cille's uncle and first cousin defeated Diarmait mac Cerbaill in 561. The early eighth-century Iona annals (AU) record that the battle was won *per orationes Coluim Cille*, through the prayers of Colum Cille, but say nothing as to its cause, nor do they ascribe any blame to the saint. Colum Cille's biographer Adomnán, writing about 700, merely refers to the battle as having occurred two years before Colum Cille's exile (Anderson 1991, 30–31). Maghnus Ó Domhnaill, writing of the Battle of Cúl Drebene in his Life of

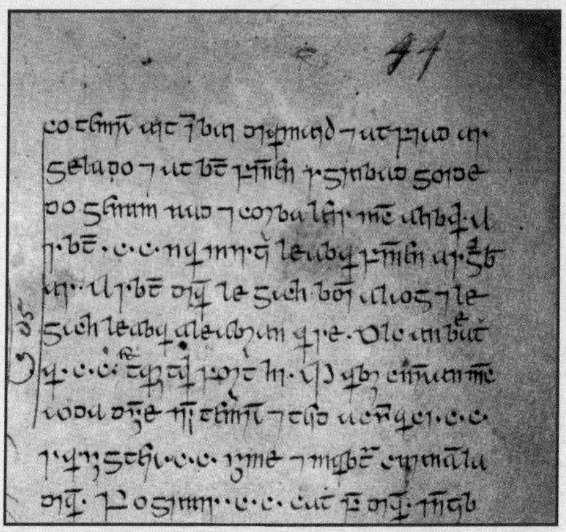

Fig. 1—Extract from RIA MS 24.P.25 (*Leabhar Chlainne Suibhne*, sixteenth century), fol. 44r, citing Diarmait mac Cerbaill's copyright ruling on the *Cathach*. (© Royal Irish Academy)

Colum Cille (O'Kelleher and Schoepperle 1918, §178; Lacey 1998, 100) at his castle in Lifford in 1532, explained the name *Cathach* (Battler or Champion) as follows:

> An Cathuch, imorro, ainm an leabhuir sin
> triasa tugadh an cath, as é is airdmhind do
> C.C. a crich Cineoil Conaill Gulban. Agus ata
> sé cumhdaigthe d'airged fa ór, ⁊ ni dleghur a
> fhoscludh. Agus da cuirther tri huaire desiul a
> timchell sluaigh Cineoil Conaill é, ag dul
> docum cat[h]a doib, is dual co ticfadh slan fa
> buaidh.

> (The Cathach, moreover, is the name of the
> book which caused that battle. It is the chief
> relic of Colum Cille in the territory of Cinél
> Conaill Gulban. And it is enshrined in a silver
> gilt box which it is not lawful to open. And
> whenever it be carried three times, turning
> towards the right, around the army of the
> Cinél Conaill when they are going into battle,
> the army usually comes back victorious.)
> (Transl. courtesy of F.J. Byrne)

The twelfth-century Latin Life of Mo Laisse of Devenish (i.e. Devenish Island) (Plummer 1910, vol. 2, 139) asserts that in view of the large numbers of men killed in the battle, the penance imposed by Mó Laisse on Colum Cille was exile. He left Ireland for Iona with twelve followers in 563 and died there on 9 June 597.[3] From Iona he founded the Hebridean island monasteries of Tiree and Hinba, the latter of which can most plausibly be identified with Canna, where there are important early Christian slabs and crosses (Campbell 1986, 5–6). It was from Iona that the Northumbrian mission was begun by Aidan with the foundation of Lindisfarne in 635. Colum Cille is credited with writing the *Altus Prosator*, a Latin poem of 23 six-line stanzas. At his death, Dallán Forgaill, 'ardollom Hérend' (Chief Poet of Ireland), composed the obscure *Amra Choluimb Chille*, an elegy of 183 lines, in which there is reference to his learning and to his interest in the Psalms:

> Gáis gluassa glé.
> Glinnsius salmu,
> sluinnsius léig libru,
> libuir ut car Cassion.

> (By his wisdom he made glosses clear.
> He fixed the Psalms,
> he made known the Books of Law,
> those books Cassian loved.) (Clancy and
> Márkus 1995, 106–8).

Adomnán's Life records several anecdotes about books and the writing of them on Iona. The saint wrote in a little hut made of wooden planks using an inkhorn (Book I, 19); on one occasion he wrote in the doorway of the hut (Book II, 16). On the day before he died he sat in his hut transcribing the psalter for the last time, stopping at the thirty-third Psalm with the famous phrase

---

[3] Dan Mc Carthy (2001) has argued that the Clonmacnoise set of annals has an internally consistent chronology that is at variance with that of the Annals of Ulster (AU) and has suggested that the death of Colum Cille took place in 593, not 597. However, the evidence of Adomnán, Bede and the majority of the Irish annals points to Sunday, 9 June 597, as the date of his death.

'Here, at the end of the page, I must stop. Let Baithene write what follows' (Book III, 23). Psalters were corrected by two pairs of eyes (Book I, 23). The account of two miracles records that books were carried from place to place in leather satchels (Book II, 8). That they were enshrined as early as Adomnán's time is suggested by the story in the same chapter of Book II. (For these and other events in the life of Colum Cille, see Reeves 1857; Anderson and Anderson 1961; Anderson 1991; Smyth 1984, 84–115; Herbert 1988; Sharpe 1995.)

When the shrine of the *Cathach* was opened by Sir William Betham, Deputy Ulster King of Arms, in 1813, he found only 58 vellum membranes of the psalter remaining, representing Psalms 30:10 to 105:13 (Betham 1826, 110–11; Lawlor 1916, 245).[4] The late Roger Powell, who rebound the manuscript in 1980, deduced from the pricking and ruling (Fig. 2) that it was bound in ten-leaf quinions, gatherings of five conjoint bifolia making twenty pages, of which five complete quinions and the greater portion of a sixth have survived.[5] Each gathering appears to have been sewn with a thread passing through three widely separated holes in the spine; Betham (1826, 110) noted that 'the sewing had almost entirely disappeared' when he first saw the manuscript. This arrangement in quinions conforms to a practice widespread, if not universal, in insular manuscripts as late at least as the Book of Armagh, written in 807. A lost eighth-century manuscript containing Old Irish saga material, the *Cín Drummo Snechtai* (of Dromsnat in County Monaghan), derived its name (Irish *cín*, from quinion) from this tradition of book-making.

The manuscript is written in a book-hand composed of confident, round letters with bold wedge serifs on the upright strokes, 'a deliberate creation out of elements of the several scripts inherited from antiquity which the earliest missionaries had brought with them' (Bieler 1963, 17). Lowe's statement that it represents 'the pure milk of Irish calligraphy' (CLA[2], xvi), is

---

[4] Psalm numbers referred to in this booklet and on the *Cathach* CD-ROM follow the Vulgate numbering, which differs slightly between Psalms 9 and 147 from that in the Authorised or King James Bible, which follows the Hebrew numbering.

[5] An extract from Roger Powell's report of 1981 on the repair and rebinding of the *Cathach*, with illustrations of the probable gatherings of the folios, is printed in Appendix 2.

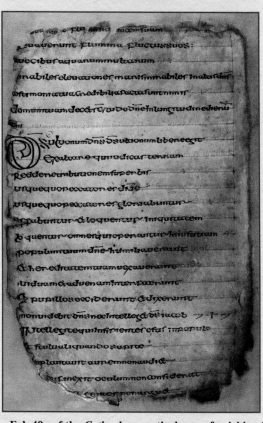

Fig. 2—Fol. 49v of the *Cathach*: a vertical row of pricking is visible at the ends of the ruled lines on the right-hand side of the folio.

often quoted; he allowed that a date as early as the time of Colum Cille is 'palaeographically possible' (CLA[2], 41). The psalms are written in brown or black ink, identified as gall, and are arranged on the page *per cola et commata* (by phrases and clauses) to facilitate reading or chanting aloud. Above each psalm is a heading written in orange in a space left for it by the scribe.

Lawlor (1916, 247–50) deduced that the minimum size of the pages was 235mm by 155mm, each pricked and ruled to take 25 lines of writing. He counted nearly 250 textual errors, most of them due to carelessness. Of 48 cases where one or more letters of a word is omitted, only 9 are corrected; over 70 corrections are made by erasure of one or more letters. He inferred that the insertion of superfluous letters, the copyist's most frequent error, was almost always detected and set right, while the omission of letters, to which he was also prone, was rarely detected. He observed that a large proportion of the corrections were made *currente calamo*, in the course of transcription, and that the manuscript was probably not compared with the exemplar after it was completed. Lawlor (1916, 250) concluded that the scribe was 'a penman of more than average excellence, who could not write rapidly but who was working at unusually high pressure when he made this transcript'.

Timothy O'Neill, a professional calligrapher, has observed (pers. comm.) that the scribe of the *Cathach* used an edged rather than a pointed quill, holding this at a fairly flat angle to the horizontal. This produced thick downstrokes and thin horizontals. The letters of the book-hand of the *Cathach* are formed by a sequence of strokes, left to right, top to bottom. Uncial (majuscule) *S* is formed of three strokes made with the pen held horizontally; *O* of two vertical strokes. The wedge serifs at the head of the verticals require an extra stroke each time and are not a feature of cursive writing, which is often characterised by signs of haste. This formal book-hand required, in O'Neill's view, a competent scribe writing in a controlled hand, fluently, without haste.

Each psalm commences with a decorative initial letter followed by a diminishing series of letters that merge into normal script (Nordenfalk 1947, 154). The initial, created by a thick black line on the vellum, is often surrounded by dotting in orange minium and has some elements filled with white lead tinged pink with madder, occasionally tinged with orange; Henry (1965, 61) noted the apposition between flat tint and dots, and the sharp definition of the lines. Commenting on the sensitivity of the artist to 'the subtle tracery of a pattern or to the sharpness of a line', she compared their attractive hesitancy to the art found on early pillars of stone. She observed that there may have been a decorated first page, now missing, which 'would have been invaluable for our knowledge of Irish illumination'. She considered that the manuscript, written well before the development of Northumbrian scriptoria, represents 'an essential landmark in the history of insular illumination'.

The *Cathach* psalter was probably kept in a *tiag*, or leather satchel, during the early centuries of its existence. It is unlikely that the manuscript would have survived to the eleventh century, when its *cumhdach* or metal shrine is believed to have been made, without the intervention of hereditary keepers or the protection of a monastic milieu guaranteed by its traditional ascription to Colum Cille.

The eponymous ancestor of the Ó Domhnaill dynasty that ruled Tír Conaill from 1200 until 1608 was Domnall, who died in 965 (AU), and whose father Éicnechán (died 906) and grandfather Dálach (died 870) were kings of Cenél Conaill. Domnall claimed descent from the fifth-century Conall, son of Niall Noígiallach (Niall of the Nine Hostages) and ancestor of Colum Cille and his successors, the abbots of Iona.[6] Dálach was of the Cenél Lugdech sept, whose home territory included the Columban sites of Gartan and Kilmacrenan. Domnall's son Conchobar is styled king of Loch Beagh at his death in 1005. In 1129 (AU; 1130 AI) Áed Ua Domnaill was burnt to death in the church of Colum Cille at Kilmacrenan: he was son of the Cathbarr Ua Domnaill who enshrined the *Cathach* and who died as king of Cenél Lugdech in 1106.

Cathbarr Ua Domnaill was son of Gilla Críst, son of Cathbarr, son of Domnall, and he was killed by his great-nephew, the son of Conn Ua Domnaill, in 1038 (AU). This son of Conn, son of Cathbarr, may have been the Tadc mac Cuinn from whom the medieval O'Donnells descended; their claim to include the second Cathbarr, son of Gilla Críst, in their ancestry is found only in a relatively late source compiled in the reign of the great Aodh Dubh Ó Domhnaill (1505–37), father of the Maghnus Ó Domhnaill who wrote the Irish Life of Colum Cille in 1532 and who was himself to rule Tír Conaill from 1537 until his deposition by his son An Calbhach in 1555 (Maghnus died on 9 February 1566).

---

[6] The Ó Domhnaill family name is hereafter referred to, at different historical periods and in variant spellings, as Ua/Uí Dom[h]naill, Ó Domhnaill or (anglicised) O'Don[n]el[l].

It is most probable that the enshrinement of the *Cathach* in a metal box (Fig. 3) took place in 1090, the year in which, according to the Clonmacnoise Annals of Tigernach (AT), Óengus Ua Domnalláin brought the relics of Colum Cille from the north:

> Minda Colaim Chille .i. Clog na Righ 7 an
> Chuillebaigh 7 in dá Sosscéla do tabairt a Tír
> Conaill 7 .uíí. fichit uínge d'airged 7
> Aenghus. H. Domnallan is se dos·fuc atuaidh.

> (The relics of Colum Cille, i.e. the Bell of the
> Kings and the Cuilebad [Flabellum] and the
> two Gospels brought from Tír Conaill, and
> seven score ounces of silver; and it was
> Óengus Ua Domnalláin who brought them
> from the north.) (trans. courtesy of F.J. Byrne)

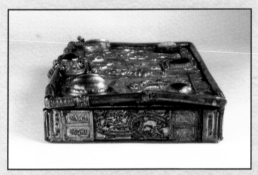

Fig. 3—Shrine of the *Cathach*: the gilt silver panel in the centre of the side of the box is part of the original eleventh-century work and features interlaced animals in the Hiberno-Norse *Ringerike* style. The lid was refurbished at a later date. (© National Museum of Ireland)

Ó Floinn (1995, 122) has suggested, following Herbert (1988, 93), that the *Cathach* was one of the 'two Gospels' referred to.

In a charter in the Book of Kells that can be dated to between 1076 and 1080, Máel Sechnaill mac Conchobair Ua Maíl Shechnaill and the coarb of Colum Cille, Domnall mac Robartaig (died 1098), granted the hermitage of Dísert Coluim Chille at Kells to God and to 'pious exiles'. In another charter, which cannot be later than 1094, Óengus Ua Domnalláin appears as confessor (*anmchara*) of Kells and also coarb of Dísert Coluim Chille, but Ferdomnach Ua Clucáin (died 1114) is coarb of Colum Cille, implying that Domnall mac Robartaig had retired from that position (Mac Niocaill 1990, 155–7). Mac Robartaig had succeeded Gilla Críst Ua Maíl Doraid, abbot of Iona, as coarb of Colum Cille in or after 1062.

The bringing of the relics from the North in 1090 suggests a deliberate policy on the part of Kells to assert its primacy over the Columban community in Ireland rather than the mere presence there of the skilled craftsman Sitric, son of Mac Áeda, whose name is inscribed on the *cumhdach*. It has been remarked that the terms of the inscription are unusual in that two patrons of the work are named. In the reading given here, the positions of rivets are marked by asterisks. Following established conventions, missing letters are given in square brackets and incomplete letters shown with a dot underneath:

> [*O]Ṛ*[*O]IT DỌ [C]Ḥ[AT]ḤB*ARR UA
> D[*O]M[*NA]ILL LASINDERN[*A]D IN
> CUMTAOH[*S]Ạ |
> 7 D*O SITT*RIUC MAC Ṃ*EIC A*EDA
> DO*RIGN[E] 7 [DO DO]M*Ṇ[ALL] M[A]C
> Ṛ[*OBA] |*
> ṚṬAIG DO COMAR[*B]A CENANSA
> LASI[N*]ḌERNAD*

(A prayer for Cathbarr Ua Domnaill who had this shrine made and for Sitric son of Mac Áeda who made [it] and for Domnall Mac Robartaig the coarb of Kells who had it made.) (trans. courtesy of F.J. Byrne)

The enshrinement may equally have been an assertion of the legitimacy of Cathbarr's claim to kingship, as the chief dynastic families of Tír Conaill from the tenth century to the end of the twelfth century were Ua Canannáin and Ua Maíl Doraid, based in the south of the territory (Gillespie 1995, 794–6, 813–14). Another battle-relic of Colum Cille's, his *cochall*, or cowl, is specifically associated in sources of the eleventh and twelfth centuries (Best and O'Brien 1967, 1298) with their ancestor Áed mac Ainmerech (killed in 598). Ua Domnaill supremacy after the reign of Éicnechán (1201–8) was firmly established by his son Domnall Mór, king of Tír Conaill and Fir Manach from 1201 to 1208.

Cathbarr's own name may have had special significance. An early hymn to Colum Cille ascribed to Adomnán and later referred to by Maghnus Ó Domhnaill is called a *cathbarr*, or helmet, in two manuscripts that derive from the lost twelfth-century Book of Glendalough (Carney 1964, xiii). The twelfth-century saga of the Death of Muirchertach Mac Erca (Nic Dhonnchadha 1964, 8) refers to the *Cathach*, in the hands of the Cenél Conaill, as one of the three battle-standards (*meirge*) of the Uí Néill, the others being the Bell of St Patrick's Testament (enshrined by Domnall Ua Lochlainn in the 1090s) and the medieval shrine known as the *Mísach* of St Cairnech of Dulane near Kells.

The Mac Robhartaigh[7] family was probably given lands at the Columban church of Drumhome (Ballymagrorty) near Ballyshannon in the thirteenth century by the Uí Dhomhnaill when that family moved to nearby Assaroe to plant the former Ua Canannáin and Ua Mael Doraid lands. It can be suggested that the *Cathach* was at Drumhome as early as the middle of the thirteenth century on the basis of a poem contained in the Book of Fenagh (Hennessy and Kelly 1875, 166–171) that mentions Drumhome and the *Cathach* manuscript, attributing the writing of it to Colum Cille. It appears that the *Cathach* was kept in a crypt under a late church in the townland of Ballymagrorty Scotch that was demolished in the nineteenth century, the ancient Ráth Cunga (Racoon) (Ó Cochláin 1968, 161), a Patrician foundation where Assicus of Elphin and Rathlin O'Birne was buried *c.* 500.

What may be an oblique reference to the *Cathach* is found in a poem written about 1230 by Giolla Brighde mac Con Midhe (Williams 1980, 18) in which there is mention of the *lúireach* (breastplate) of Colum Cille; described as the words of Colum Cille in battle (*briathra Colaim Chille i gcath*), this may echo the early hymn to Colum Cille, ascribed to Adomnán, which is called a *cathbarr* or helmet. The later poem was written in praise of

---

[7] Mac Robhartaigh is the modern Irish spelling of mac Robartaig; the name is anglicised, in variant spellings, as Roarty, McRoarty, McGroarty, Magroarty.

Domhnall Mór Ó Domhnaill, king of Tír Conaill and Fír Manach from 1208 to 1241. His line continued through his son Domhnall Óg (1258–61), grandson Aodh (1281–1333), great-grandson Seán (1362–80) and great-great-grandson Toirdealbhach an Fhíona (1380–1422). The line is further traced through Toirdealbhach an Fhiona's son Niall Garbh (1422–39). Of these figures, Toirdealbhach an Fhíona, who appointed the Ó Cléirigh family as historians to the Ó Domhnaill family, had the kind of prominence that makes him a likely candidate to have refurbished the *Cathach* with a new top plate that resembles fourteenth-century work on the shrine known as the *Domhnach Airgid* (Armstrong and Lawlor 1918).

The *Cathach* was captured and its *maor* (keeper) Mac Robhartaigh slain at the battle of Bealach Buidhe near Boyle in 1497, when the Ó Domhnaill family were defeated by MacDermot of Moylurg. It was brought to the battle of Fearsad Mór (near Letterkenny) fought between O'Neill and O'Donnell in 1567, when its custodian, another Mac Robhartaigh, was slain (AFM). Colgan (1647, 495) wrote that in his time the *Cathach* was kept at Ballymagrorty in the parish of Drumhome. It was carried away from Tír Conaill by Colonel Daniel O'Donel of Ramelton, who followed King James II to France after the Battle of the Boyne in 1690. O'Donel had the *cumhdach* refurbished and inscribed on the Continent in 1723; he also engraved the O'Donel arms on a semi-circular projection midway along the front of the base (as described by Armstrong in Lawlor 1916, 395–6). The coat of arms is a version similar to that granted to O'Donel in a certificate of arms by the Athlone Pursuivant at the Jacobite court at St Germain-en-Laye, James Terry, in 1709 (Hayes 1949, 296–7). O'Donel died on 7 July 1735, leaving a widow and a fourteen-year-old daughter.

George Petrie (OSL, 216) records that before his death Daniel O'Donel deposited the *Cathach* in a monastery, which can plausibly be identified as the convent of the Irish Benedictine nuns at Ypres in Flanders (modern Belgium) (Herity 2000, 462). This convent had close connections with the court of James III: a Mr O'Donnell was appointed confessor there in 1701 by the Dowager Queen Mary (Historical Manuscripts Commission 1902, 161). It can be assumed that some doubts as to who the legitimate heir to the title 'The O'Donnell' might be and who would therefore be entitled to the keepership of the *Cathach* led

O'Donel to take the unusual step of depositing the manuscript there; he stipulated in writing that it should be given up to the chief of the clan when applied for (OSL, 216).

It appears that the reliquary was seen at the 'monastery' by Father Prendergast, Parish Priest and titular Augustinian Abbot of Cong from 1795, who, it has been implied, was a seminarian at nearby St Omer (Wilde 1867, 174n.), probably in the 1760s. He informed Sir Neal O'Donel of Newport, County Mayo, who had bought the former abbey lands at Cong in 1780 (Ó Cochláin 1968, 171). Sir Neal applied for the *Cathach* as chief of the family but was required to provide a certificate attested by Sir William Betham, Deputy Ulster King of Arms, to support his claim; the *Cathach* was handed over in 1813 to his brother Connel O'Donel, who was then on the continent (OSL, 216).

Betham (1826, 109–10) described in his *Irish antiquarian researches* how he examined the metal shrine with the ready permission of 'its present possessor, Connel O'Donell, Esq.'. Disregarding 'injunctions and threats of ignorance, which for more than a century had hermetically sealed it up, under an idea that it contained the bones of St. Columkill himself…the box was opened and examined in the presence of Sir Capel Molyneux, Mr O'Donell, and myself, without any extraordinary, or supernatural occurrence…'. Inside he found the manuscript, covered on one side with 'a thin piece of board covered with red leather, very like that with which eastern MSS. are bound'. As folio 58v, the last surviving page of the manuscript, bears traces of abrasion, probably from contact with the metal of the shrine, it seems likely that the cover of red leather on board had lain at the front of the surviving membranes.

The following scenario can be proposed to reconcile various accounts of the return of the *Cathach* to Ireland—Betham's (1826, 20–21, 109–10, 189), Petrie's (OSL, 216), O'Donovan's (AFM, 2400) and O'Curry's (1861, 331). Continual war between 1802 and 1813 made access to Flanders difficult. Sir Capel Molyneux, son-in-law of Sir Neal O'Donel, and his wife, Margaret, had sought out the *Cathach* at a monastery in Flanders during the short-lived peace that followed the Treaty of Amiens in 1802. As Petrie has recorded, proof was required of the right of the O'Donels of Newport to keepership of the relic before it would be released. In 1805 William Betham came to Dublin and later became Deputy Ulster King of Arms; he was knighted in

1812. The certificate 'To All and Singular' at the end of an O'Donnell genealogy, now in the Royal Irish Academy and attested by Betham on 30 September 1813, is probably the one mentioned by Petrie as the authority that Connel O'Donel required to claim and acquire the *Cathach* from the monastery in Flanders late in that year. A copy of this genealogy and its proofs in MS G.O. 169 of the Genealogical Office, Dublin, is also dated 30 September 1813. It would appear that the shrine came to Ireland only after this genealogy was made. The opening of the shrine and the discovery of the psalter, which Betham describes as having taken place in his study in Blackrock, County Dublin, in the presence of Mr Connel O'Donel and Sir Capel Molyneux, can be dated to 1813 by the Bill of Complaint filed against Betham for opening the shrine by Dame Mary O'Donel on 30 April 1814; these events apparently took place in the last months of 1813. Betham first tested his hypothesis that the shrine contained a manuscript by passing a 'slender wire' through a small opening, with which he rubbed the edges of the vellum leaves (Lawlor 1916, 244 nn 2, 3). This scenario requires that the drawings of the top and base of the shrine that appear in both of Betham's manuscript genealogies were probably added later.

The initials of the *Cathach*

Each of the surviving psalms in the *Cathach* has a rubric or heading of up to three lines written in orange minium in a space left for it by the scribe; sometimes the words are spread out to fill the space, sometimes the writing is closely crowded, occasionally it overruns the space allotted (Lawlor 1916, 252). Beneath the heading, the text of the psalm begins with an ornamented initial followed by up to three further ornamented letters (Fig. 4). Unlike those in classical manuscripts, these initials are placed within the block of psalm text, some extending as many as six lines down, some extending upwards into the text of the heading. The initials also assume an intimate relationship with the text through a series of diminishing intermediate letters. The fact that many of the 150 psalms begin with one of the same small group of letters presented a formidable challenge to the inventiveness of the Irish scribe, who wished each ornamented initial to be an original and unique creation. As Pächt (1986, 51) has observed, letters are symbols that must be understood clearly, and there is

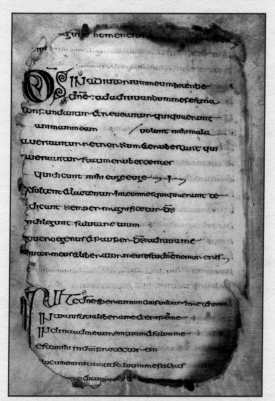

Fig. 4—Fol. 30v of the *Cathach*, showing rubrics and decorated initials of Psalms 69 and 70.

therefore a limit beyond which ornamentation should not be carried.

The great majority of these initials are based on the uncial, or majuscule, forms of the letters, and the artist wishing to devise ornamental versions was both limited and liberated by their forms. Sixty-five initials have survived, intact or fragmentary (see Figs 5–10 for a selection of the initials). Traces of a dotted outline in minium, which in most cases has retained its orange colour but in a few has turned brown, can now be discerned on up to 47 of these, most of them well-preserved examples. Painting in the body of the letter in a white colour tinged with pink is more difficult to discern with certainty but seems to occur in 35 initials, including two instances where a light red, possibly minium, is used. There is more room for doubt in the early folios of the

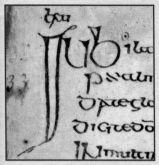

Fol. 26r

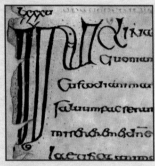

Fol. 43v

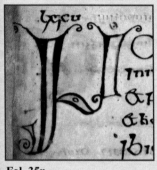

Fol. 35r

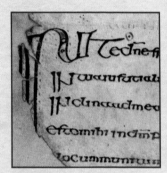

Fol. 30v

Fig. 5—Initial *I* (fols 26r, 43v); initial *N* (fol. 35r); *N* not in initial position (fols 30v, 43v). On fol. 43v *INCL*: *I* and *N* are both surrounded by dotting. On fol. 30v *IN te dñe*: *I* and *N* are surrounded by dotting; cross-member of *N* shows clear traces of orange.

manuscript, up to about fol. 28v; it may be that the blotting-paper used by Betham (1826, 111) to separate the folios after the discover of the manuscript has obscured a greater proportion of the features of these early folios. The limited technical resources available to Lawlor (1916, 252) led him to count only 20 initials with traces of colour in the body of the letter and 42 outlined with orange dots. Where the half-uncial letter forms are used, the motivation may have been a desire for diversity; alternatively, this form may have presented the artist with a more suitable model for ornamentation, as in the case of the letter *B*. It appears that an edged quill of the type used for writing the book-hand of the text was also used for the thick down-strokes; here too it was held at a fairly flat angle to the horizontal, as is evidenced in the alignment of the thin oblique strokes of the initial *O* of fol. 14v. Whereas such initials as those on fols 4r and 13r seem to have been formed with a single downstroke, many other verticals were doubled to achieve the desired thickness; this was also achieved by filling between two outer lines, as in the lower left-hand member of the initial *U* on fol. 35v.

Those initials that are based on upright columns necessarily depart little from the classic form of the letter: they include the five examples of initial *I* (fols 4r, 11v, 26r, 30v, 43v), the two of initial *N* (fols 6r, 35r) and the six of initial *Q* (fols 11r, 18r, 32v, 40r, 42v, 48r). Initial *I* is tall, up to five line spaces in height; it is composed of two verticals made with the quill, between which an open space is left for painting; it narrows from top to bottom and has a slight freehand curve; the top is finished with a spiral-ended yoke, Duval's *accolade* (Duval 1977, 284), the lower end with a thin tail tending left. The treatment is freehand, the shape influenced by the wedge-shaped serif found on smaller versions of the letter, and with curvilinear embellishments at the ends.

In the two examples of initial *N* a longer left-hand vertical column five line spaces in height is treated in the same manner as initial *I* but with elaborations of the lower end based on Irish La Tène motifs.[8] The right-hand vertical column is shorter, with spiral elaborations at the upper end; in each of the two initial *N*s

---

[8] The La Tène flourished in central Europe in the late Iron Age and came to pre-Christian Ireland *c*. 300 BC. Its distinctive curvilinear style was evident in the stone and metal work, weaponry and decorative art of this period and also carried on into the early Christian period in Ireland.

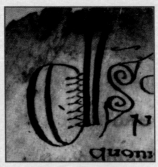

Fol. 42r

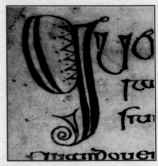

Fol. 11r

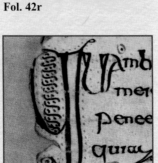

Fol. 32v

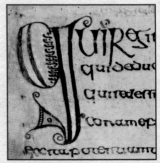

Fol. 40r

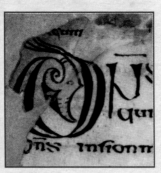

Fol. 52v

Fig. 6—Half-uncial *D* (fol. 42r); initial *Q* (fols 11r, 32v, 40r); initial *D* with animal head (fol. 52v). On fol. 42r *D* and *S* are both surrounded by faint dotting. On fol. 11r see lower left of spiral in *Q* where doubled pen line can be seen in magnification. On fol. 32v each of the first four letters (*QUAM*) is surrounded by dotting. On fol. 40r initial *Q* is surrounded by faint dotting; a zoomorphic impression is created by the eye-dot in the embellishment at the lower end. On fol. 52v initial *D* is surrounded by dots. Note the *trompe l'oeil* effect created by the neck of the beast.

it is joined to the taller left-hand column by a curved, eyed fish-like element with spiral tail. The uncial *N* of *Inclina* (fol. 43v) is treated similarly: its S-curved, fish-like element joins the base of the shorter right-hand column to the head of the longer left-hand one and has a collar as well as an eye. The columns in the *N* of *In te dñe* (fol. 30v) are joined in the same manner with an S-curved fish, eyed and collared, partly painted in orange. These versions of *N* are forerunners of the more elaborate version of Codex Ambr. S 45 sup., p. 2 (Henry 1950, fig. 1; Henderson 1987, 25–8) and Durham MS A.II.10, both dated to the early seventh century, where this fish has developed into an intertwined double-headed beast (Henry 1965, pl. 61). As Henry put it:

> The extreme importance of the
> Cathach…comes from the fact that it allows
> us to grasp what the decoration of manuscripts
> was before the contacts with the Continent had
> become closer, and much before the
> development of the Northumbrian scriptoria.
> (Henry 1965, 61)

The upright column of each of the five substantially intact *Q*s (fols 11r, 32v, 40r, 42v, 48r) is similar to the uprights of *I* and *N*. In one case (fol. 48r) it has a solid body and zoomorphic counter-curve to the spiral tail; the upper end of the column has a half-yoke embellishment (Duval's *pseudo-accolade*) similar to a flourish found on some of the initials of the sixth-century Laurentian manuscript of Orosius, Plutarch 65 (Nordenfalk 1947, 153–5, figs. 10, 11, 13). In some cases the ovoid element, formed by a pair of curved lines made with a broad quill, has a narrow vertical open space intended to be painted. Each has a filler motif in the open field within the oval, either a dotted chevron—a v-shaped ornamentation (fols 11r, 42v)—or a dotted chain (fols 32v, 40r, 48r) like that forming the frame of the cross-ornamented page of the Codex Usserianus Primus (Trinity College, Dublin) (Henry 1965, pl. 58), a manuscript assigned by Lowe (CLA[2], 42) to the beginning of the seventh century. The two letters *D* that follow the half-uncial form (fols 27r, 42r) are made in similar fashion to the *Q*s but with a plainer treatment of the base of the column. One (fol. 27r) has a dotted chain filler, the other a chevron.

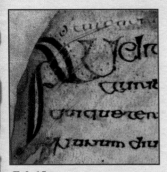

Fol. 15v

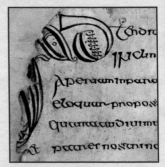

Fol. 36v

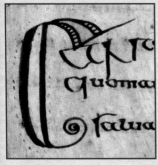

Fol. 52r

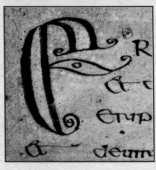

Fol. 22r

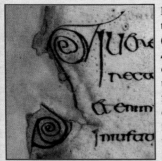

Fol. 21v

Fig. 7—Initial *A* (fols 15v, 36v) together with metalwork technique (fol. 52r); *C* (fol. 52r), *E* (fol. 22r) and *S* (fol. 21v). On fol. 15v the uprights of the letter *A* are filled with paint; the first two letters are dotted. On fol. 36v a very elaborate initial *A* is constructed of zoomorphic elements including a beast partially shown at the bottom left. On fol. 52r initial *C* has an upper element reminiscent of metalwork. The outlines of this bold initial are dotted. On fol. 22r the bold shape of the initial *C* is adapted to form an *E* by the addition of a fish, swimming. On fol. 21v initial *S* and many of the letters that follow it are decorated with dotting.

Five *C*s (fols 34v, 51r, 52r, 56v, 58r) and six *E*s (fols 13r, 22r, 23v, 25r, 27r, 41r) survive as decorative initials. Each shaft is based on a vertical line set on the right within a thicker curved crescent, leaving a narrow space between; these lines cross over at the top to form the downturn at the top right of the letter, embellished with a spiral-ended yoked flourish, biased towards the right. At the base they taper to a small spiral in all cases except one (fol. 51r), where the yoke of the upper end of the *C* is repeated in miniature at the lower end. The *E*s have an extra member in the form of a tiny fish as the middle arm of the letter, two of which (fols 22r, 23v) have an eye-circle. The only initial *F* (fol. 44r) is of a similar form, with an upper curved member springing to the right from the top right-hand corner of a paired-line column and terminating in an asymmetrical yoke. The lower horizontal member of this *F* is also a fish-like curve.

The fragmentary *T* of fol. 25v follows the half-uncial form and ends in a small, tight spiral. It is constructed of two pairs of curved lines, each pair bounding an open space. The space is filled by a row of dots, as in La Tène metalwork. The only surviving initial *O* (fol. 14v) is of simple construction, drawn with pairs of lines bounding an open space at the upper right and lower left. The *m* of the word *Omnes* and the first four letters of the first word on the next line, *iubilate*, fill its inner space, suggesting that the initial *O* was made first in this case. Another *o* (fol. 34v), not in initial position and drawn with a thick line, is filled with a dotted chain motif down its centre.

The remaining initials, *D, B, U, S, M* and *A*, lend themselves to a curvilinear mode more in keeping with La Tène forms and style. In eighteen uncial initial *D*s (fols 7v, 8v, 12r, 14r, 18v, 19r, 23r, 24v, 30v, 39v, 41v, 44r, 47r, 49r, 49v, 51v, 52v, 53v) the basic circle or oval is usually two-and-a-half line spaces in depth, with the curved triangular ascender extending as much as two line spaces above and to the left. Double lines with open spaces within form both vertical sides of the circular element; where the triangular ascender is preserved it often has a curved yoke flourish at the end. In one case (fol. 19r) the ascender, itself a pelta, or representation of a whale's tail, contains a second, tiny, painted pelta; in another (fol. 44v) it merges into what appears to be a spiral-ended cross form. In all cases there is an attempt to fill the open circular space: eight *D*s (fols 7v, 14r, 19r, 23r, 24v, 41v, 44v, 51v) and a possible ninth (fol. 47r) have dotted chain motifs;

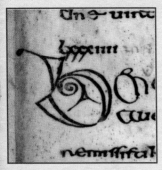

Fol. 43r

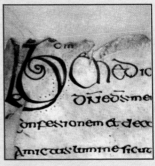

Fol. 55v

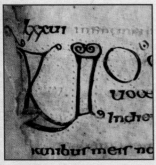

Fol. 35v

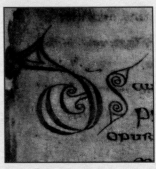

Fol. 12r

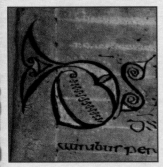

Fol. 19r

Fig. 8—Initial *B* (fols 43r, 55v); initial *U* (fol. 35v); uncial *D* (fols 12r, 19r). On fol. 43r, traces of dotting are visible around the first letters of *BENEDIXISTI*. On fol. 55v, dots outline the *B*, which has two trumpet-curves meeting at a lentoid, bottom left. On fol. 35v there are traces of paint in the right-hand upright, which ends in a double inturned spiral design at the upper end; the orange dotting is well marked. On fol. 12r the letter *D* is built on the fulcrum of a pelta. On fol. 19r the use of paint to fill major spaces in the *D* and to highlight details like the pelta (top left) and the triangles at the ends of the letter *S* is well demonstrated. The faintest traces of dotting remain around the outer edge of the initial.

three (fols 8v, 39v, 52v) have spirals—one (fol. 52v) incorporates part of a stylised animal head, the other two end in La Tène trumpet counter-curves; three further examples (fols 18v, 30v, 49v) have simple La Tène trumpets; two (fols 12r, 53v) have peltas. The most elaborate example (fol. 19r) has a pair of trumpets meeting at a lentoid, or lens-shaped element, in the right-hand side of the circle and a similar angled expansion in the pair of lines opposite, echoing a feature of the treatment of initials *B* and *U* described below.

Each of the five decorated initial *B*s (fols 3r, 43r, 48v, 54v, 55v) consists of a lower circular element, drawn with paired lines on the upper right and lower left, with a wide vertical trumpet-shaped ascender; in three cases (fols 43r, 48v, 55v) the ascender is elaborated by a yoke rising above it to the left or right. Four (fol. 43r, 48v, 54v, 55v) were designed with a distinctive sharp angle towards the lower left-hand side, in one case (fol. 55v) marked by a lentoid. While this form can be seen as influenced by the half-uncial letter, which has a straight vertical left-hand member like the modern lower-case letter *b*, the concept underlying the structure is equally plausibly a design formed of three La Tène elements: a pair of trumpets meeting in the lower left-hand corner, e.g. at the lentoid of fol. 55v, and a spiral-ended crescent closing the oval element of the letter at the top right. In three cases the space in the circular element is filled with decoration: a dotted chain (fol. 54v), a further trumpet-like motif, counter-curved and partially surviving (fol. 3r), and a triskele (fol. 43r).

The three *U*s (fols 33v, 35v, 50v) are based on a vertical columnar member on the right and a curvilinear member on the left. In two cases (fols 33v and 50v) the upper terminals of each column have a spiral-ended yoke-like flourish that is biased to the right; the third has a symmetrical pair of inturned spirals. Each column also has a yoked embellishment at the lower end. The bottom left side of one example (fol. 35v), and probably of a second (fol. 50v), is angled and, like the letter *B*, trumpet-based in concept.

S is represented twice as a decorative initial (fols 21v, 28v) and elsewhere as a decorative letter not in initial position. In each case it appears that the uncial form was used, based on a pair of spirals each with a triangular projection ending in a long flourish, like versions of *S* in the Ambrosian Codex S 45 sup. (Henry 1950,

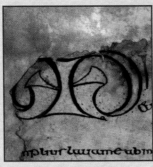

Fol. 17v

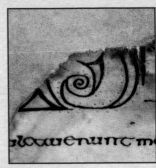

Fol. 20v

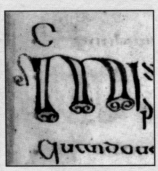

Fol. 53r

Fig. 9—Initial *M* (fols 17v, 20v, 53r). In the *M* on fol. 17v the central column and the curved upright element on the right are painted; orange dotting outlines the letter; the circles are compass-drawn— the central perforation left by the dividers shows on fol. 17r. The *M* on fol. 20v also appears to be compass-drawn; a scratched line made by the dividers shows between the line of dots and the inner edge of the curved line, bottom right. On fol. 53r, the initial *M* stands on three pairs of apposed spirals and is outlined with orange dotting; a number of curved quill-strokes can be seen in the far right-hand upright element.

fig. 10; see further discussion of this manuscript on pp 29 and 37 below). The upper terminal of the fragmentary example of *S* on fol. 28v is filled with traces of what can be reconstructed as a cross with expanded terminals (see Fig. 11a below). The triangular appendage above is conceived as two trumpets meeting at a lentoid that is filled with three dots in line.

There are five surviving examples of *M* in initial position (fols 17v, 20v, 21r, 45r, 53r). In three monumental constructions of the letter (fols 17v, 20v, 21r), and possibly in a fourth fragmentary *M* of the same type (fol. 45r), the uncial form is elaborated in the curvilinear idiom of Irish La Tène. A central column with concave sides supports on either side circular forms based on compass-drawn circles with pairs of vertically-set curved lines enclosing a narrow painted space. Within the circles of fol. 21r a pair of spirals is formed, the counter-curve emerging from each spiral swelling to a lentoid between two trumpet curves. The design of the *M* of fol. 20v is similar, while the *M* on fol. 17v has a simpler design in which the outer elements curve around into the centre of each circle to meet the convex mouth of a simple trumpet. The example on fol. 53r, the half-uncial initial *M* of Psalm 100, is a brilliantly simple version of the letter with zoomorphic overtones, a playful three-footed creation shod with symmetric double spirals and with an S-curved tail.

Two initial *A*s (fols 15v, 36v), each based on the uncial form, are elaborate structures. Both are formed of two major fish-like curved elements, each enclosing an open space between curved lines, the longer, lower, vertical element joining the upper, diagonal one about half-way along its underside. These elements are joined by a third, tiny, fish-like curve that closes the *A* near the base of the diagonal fish above. Each *A* is bounded by thick lines: in the less elaborate one (fol. 15v) each main element consists of a single pair of lines with painting between, the lower end of each ending in a flourish; the more elaborate *A* (fol. 36v) has double paired lines defining the two major elements, with thicker lines on the inside of the upper element, which also has an eye-circle and a collar. An open-mouthed 'beast' can be reconstructed, curling round from the lowermost extremity of the letter.

Two further fragmentary crosses associated with initial letters have been detected in the *Cathach* since Lawlor's study. Traces of the upper limb and right arm of the first are discernible on fol. 28v in the surviving upper fragment of the initial letter *S* of *Salvum* in

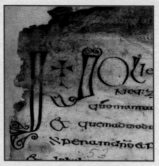

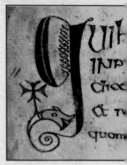

Fol. 6r

Fol. 48r

Fol. 50v

Fig. 10—Equal-armed crosses standing on uprights in and ⟨of⟩ initials on fols 6r, 48r and 50v.

Psalm 68 (Fig. 11a), where two characteristic pointed curves can be viewed as part of a tiny cross that is very similar to those depicted on fols 48r and 50v. The second cross (Fig. 11b), noted by Roth (1979, 68), is more fully preserved: it forms an extension of the end of the initial *D* of *Domine Deus* in Psalm 87 (fol. 44v). It has an expanded arm like those of the other crosses but appears to have been surmounted at the upper end of the shaft by a pair of inturned spirals (like those of the initial *U* on fol. 35v). These spirals are now separated from the head by a tear in the

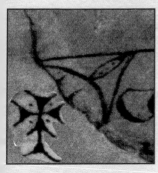

Fol. 28v

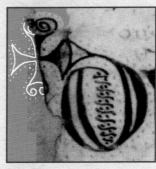

Fol. 44v

Fig. 11—Partially-defined crosses in initials: fol. 28v—probable remains of cross with expanded terminals in initial *S* of *Salvum*, with cross from fol. 50v inset for comparison; fol. 44v—equal-armed cross with inturned spiral scrolls at head and probably at the foot shown with tentative reconstruction in white.

parchment; a curve, lower right, suggests that there was originally a pair of similar spirals at the lower end of the shaft. Small dots in the two remaining cantons probably belong to a set of four, as in fol. 50v.

The main inspiration in the design of many of the initials is Irish La Tène, freehand and lively, occasionally playful. Lentoid and lobeate swellings, the triple-dot motif, trumpet ends, curve and counter-curve, peltae and spiral ends (simple or at the ends of a yoked motif) and Duval's *accolade* are almost universal. The theory that Celtic metalwork influenced the design of the initials is strongly supported by the occurrence of background hachuring or dotting in fols 25v, 30v, 40r, 48r and 52r as well as the triple-dot motifs of fols 7v, 14v, 23v, 33v and the initial *D* of fol. 52v. These triangular triple-dot arrangements in orange repeat a motif found in the free spaces of the design of a pagan Celtic scabbard-plate from the river Bann (Raftery 1983, 103–4) and are also found in the Bobbio manuscripts and later manuscripts like the books of Durrow, Lindisfarne and Kells.

The use of compasses, well known in the pre-Christian metalwork tradition, is evidenced in the design of two initial *M*s, fols 17v and 21r (Fig. 12). The centre points of the two circles in the *M* of fol. 21r are marked by dots immediately above the spiral in each (Fig. 12b). On the verso of the folio each of these dots is matched by a smaller one. Circles described on these as centres extend from the edges of the central pillar to the inner of the two lines marking the upright crescents of the *M*. This observation has been confirmed by Mr Anthony Cains (pers. comm.), Head of Conservation at the Library, Trinity College, Dublin, who has discerned under magnification perforations marked by these dots and scratched lines under the ink at points along the circumference of both circles. These marks can be explained by the use of a pair of dividers, an item of equipment that would have been commonplace in a scriptorium and that was used for the pricking and ruling of each gathering of this manuscript. The centre point of the similar, though fragmentary, initial *M* on fol. 17v (Fig. 12a) are visible on the verso of the page and match the spot where the curved line meets the wedge of the pelta in each circle. A circle described on the point of the intact right-hand circle runs from the edge of the central pillar to the outer line of the upright crescent on the right. It appears that both *M*s were designed on symmetrical pairs of compass-drawn circles that were so faintly marked that they can now be barely discerned. On fol. 20v an arc of a circle etched immediately to the right of the line of dots inside the inner right-hand curved line suggests the use of dividers in the laying-out of this *M* too. The *Cathach* thus looks back towards a design technique well known in Irish La Tène metalwork and forward to a later manuscript tradition in which designs based on the use of compasses continue the earlier traditions (Henry 1965, 206–24).

A separate, restricted set of exotic influences comes from early Christian art: manuscript conventions are represented in the forms of the initials themselves, in the Coptic dotting surrounding them and in chain and chevron filler patterns. The single spiral extension at the base of the right-hand column of the initial *U* of fol. 35v may derive from symmetrical paired spiral extensions like those at the ends of the arms of the Coptic ankh

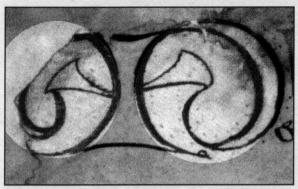

Fol. 17v

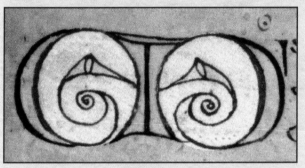

Fol. 21r

Fig. 12—Compass-drawn designs for initial *M* on fols 17v and 21r. The basic compass-drawn circles are shown in a lighter shade in each case.

of the Glazier Codex of *c.* AD 400 (Bober 1967, fig. 1). One of the five crosses that intrude into the design of a number of initials has paired symmetric spirals at least at the upper end of the shaft (fol. 44v); the others are of a simpler type with flaring terminals. A design element also greatly favoured by the scribe is a simple, fluid fish motif, often eyed, occasionally with a collar, the early Christian ιχθύς, which is rendered in a more developed form in the Bobbio manuscripts Ambrosian I 61 sup. and S 45 sup. This last manuscript, Atalanus's, also has the triple-dot motif at the foot of the column of the initial *P* and on the body of the 'fish' (Henry 1950, fig. 20*b*, *c*). In the *Cathach* this fish is frequently used as the cross-member of the letters *E*, *F* and *N* and is the basic design element in the two examples of initial *A*. The zoomorphic eye in the left-hand crescent of the *D* on fol. 51v also suggests a fish of this family. In just a few cases, fols 48r and 52v, the 'fish' is given a characteristic open beast-mouth. Is it possible to interpret these as dolphins?

These two sources, pagan Celtic and early Christian, contribute to the design of two contrasting sets of letters, one broadly columnar, the other broadly curvilinear. The *N*, its bold uprights joined by a fish cross-member, is typical of the first group, the compass-based *M*, with its trumpet, spiral and triskele fillers, of the second. Almost every initial is informed by a Celtic style, freehand, tending to the curvilinear, with asymmetric curved elaborations. The Christian fish, often simplified, is incorporated in a fluid Celtic rhythm, a feature most clearly visible in the design of both initial *A*s. In a *trompe l'oeil* detail typical of Irish Celtic art, the neck of the collared fish-beast in the initial *D* of *DÑS* on fol. 52v disappears into the void as the eye follows it outwards. Of all the manuscripts of early date from Ireland or Irish centres on the Continent, the *Cathach* shows in its initials the greatest influence of the Celtic style.

Comparanda in stone and other media for crosses in the *Cathach*

A distinctive addition to three of the decorative initials of the *Cathach* is a tiny cross with wide expanded terminals ending in points, each standing on a stem with a greatly expanded foot. One stands within the *N* of *Noli*, the first word of Psalm 36 (fol. 6r), a second stands behind the head of a fishy beast forming part of the initial *Q* of *Qui habitat*, Psalm 90 (fol. 48r), a third, with dots in each of the four cantons, sits inside the *U* of *Uenite* at the beginning of Psalm 93 (fol. 50v). A parallel for the combination of cross and dolphin on fol. 48r can be found in the Coptic world (at Armant, Egypt), in a Latin cross with expanded ends shown behind the head of a fish depicted with mouth widely splayed; this stone panel (Fig. 13) is dated to the fifth or sixth century (Badawy 1978, 186, fig. 3.140). The discovery of two further crosses (fols 28v, 44v) is noted above (see Fig. 11), the second of these being a more elaborate form apparently with inturned spirals.

Very similar crosses with expanded terminals ornament the paired terminals of four penannular brooches in the National

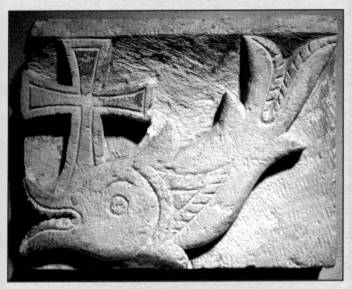

Fig. 13—Latin cross and Coptic fish from Armant, Egypt (Musée du Louvre, Paris). (© Photo RMN—B. Hatala)

Museum of Ireland (Fig. 14a–d). One of these is from County Westmeath (Fig. 14a), the other three are from unknown locations in Ireland (Haseloff 1990, 158). Two of those found at unknown locations are depicted standing on stems like those in the *Cathach* crosses (Fig. 14b, d). Duignan (1973) has reported a pair of broadly similar crosses pattée (i.e. with expanded terminals) a little over 3mm wide at either end of an *S*-scroll and within a curved rectangular band, presumably originally enamelled, on a bronze hand-pin from Treanmacmurtagh Bog in County Sligo (Fig. 14e), which she assigns to her Class IIIb. A similar stamped design on an imported pottery dish from the monastery of Tintagel in Cornwall is discussed below (p. 36).

A latchet-fastener from Ireland noted by Wilde (1861, 566–7, W.491) and dated to the fifth or sixth century has a six-petalled marigold at the centre of its disk, and the designs between the petals have the same cusped expansion at the outer ends and the same narrowing profile as the limbs of the crosses pattée on the terminals of the pennannular brooches drawn by Haseloff; the whole design of the centre of the disk is surrounded by a single incised line arranged in swags with triple-dot motifs at the points. Cross and marigold are closely related designs in early Christian

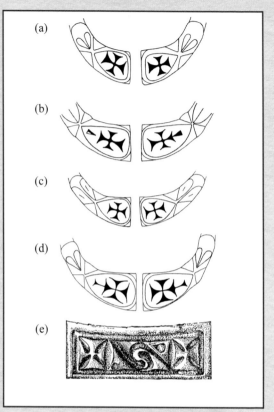

Fig. 14—Cross-ornamented terminals of penannular brooches: (a) County Westmeath; (b), (c), (d) Ireland (after Haseloff 1990); (e) detail of hand-pin from Treanmacmurtagh Bog, Sligo (after Duignan 1973).

Ireland, the one often appearing as the obverse of the other, as on a great prehistoric standing stone at Killeen in County Mayo (Herity 1995b, 235, pl. 3) and at the centre of the carpet page (fol. 85v) of the Book of Durrow.

In stone there are excellent comparanda: on a broken slab from the fifth-century foundation of St Mochaoi of Nendrum in Strangford Lough, County Down (Fig. 15a); on a boulder, part of a prehistoric burial monument at Knockane on the Dingle peninsula in County Kerry (Herity 1995b, 240–1, pl. 5.3) (Fig. 15b); and within a penannular cartouche with spiral ends on a boulder at the ecclesiastical site of Kilvickadownig at the west end of the same peninsula (Cuppage *et al.* 1986, 327, fig. 196) (Fig. 15c), where the cross stands on a stem like those of the *Cathach*. Another closely comparable cross on stem within a circular cartouche is carved on a boulder in the early ecclesiastical site at Maumanorig on the same peninsula (Cuppage *et al.* 1986, 332–3, fig. 201a) (Fig. 15d); here an ogham inscription belonging to the later post-syncope series and engraved in an unusual fashion on a curved stem-line may have been added later than the elaborate cross—Macalister (1945, 186–8) has read the inscription as *ANM COLMAN AILITHIR* ('the name of Colman the pilgrim').

A similar tiny crosslet with characteristic expanded ends is deeply engraved within a circle on a small water-worn boulder, apparently a prayer-stone or so-called 'cursing-stone', in the oratory of Senach's island foundation of Illauntannig, one of the Maharees group of islands, opposite Kilshannig, off the north coast of the Dingle peninsula (Fig. 16). A simple carving with similar expanded ends existed at Conwal in Donegal (Lacy *et al.* 1983, 258, fig. 136, pl. 36). Henry (1951, 67, 69, fig. 2) has compared the Latin cross with expanded terminals standing on a short stem depicted on her Pillar 12 on top of the Bailey Mór on

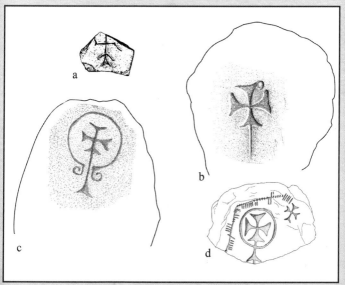

Fig. 15—Cross-engraved slabs: (a) Nendrum, (b) Knockane, (c) Kilvickadownig, (d) Maumanorig (after Cuppage *et al.* 1986).

the island of Inishkea North, off the Mullet peninsula in Mayo, with the cross-on-stem depicted on fol. 48r (Psalm 90) of the *Cathach*. A similar equal-armed cross with widely expanded terminals on the arms and shaft stands in relief on a pillar and slight base on the architrave of the doorway of the church at Clonamery in County Kilkenny. This has been compared to Armenian and Georgian crosses of the fifth to seventh centuries (Richardson 1987, 134–5).

This distinctive form of the cross was apparently widespread in Ireland, being found in counties Kerry, Westmeath, Mayo, Sligo, Donegal and Down, and is associated with early monastic foundations like Nendrum. It was particularly well known in the non-Patrician south-west (Herity 1995b, 252). Its occurrence on penannular brooches (an early form derived from Roman brooches), in a cognate form on a latchet, on a hand-pin and carved on stone slabs and pillars at ecclesiastical sites associated with early saints of the fifth and sixth centuries suggests that the models for these crosses could have been introduced substantially before 600 and may well have been in fashion

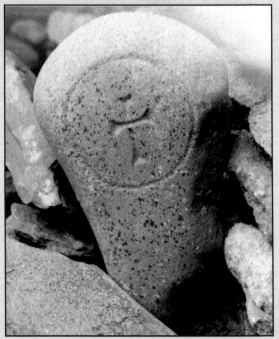

Fig. 16—Illauntannig prayer-stone with engraved cross.

throughout the sixth century, in the second half of which Colum
Cille flourished. The dominance of Irish La Tène motifs and style
in the ornamentation of the initials of the *Cathach* compared with
the scarcity of elements introduced from the Christian world
outside Ireland supports this assessment.

An equal-armed cross on a stem engraved on a stone slab
located near St Columba's Church on Inishkea North (Fig. 17),
Henry's Slab 5 (Henry 1945, 145, Pl. XXVIII, bottom right), has
decorative terminals resembling those found on some of the
Cathach initials. Here the solid ends of the arms, shaft and foot of
the stand are decorated by adding a wide yoke terminating in a
tiny spiral at either end, not unlike Duval's *accolade*, as found on
the *E* of *Eripe* on fol. 22r (Psalm 58) and the *N* of *Notus* on fol.
35r (Psalm 75). A Latin cross standing on a pedestal between two
globes on a Byzantine medallion dated to the first half of the fifth
century, now in the Walters Art Gallery in Baltimore (Haseloff

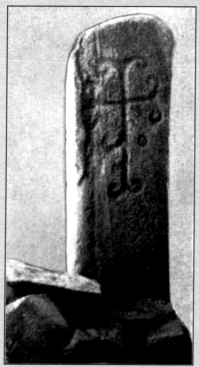

**Fig. 17—Engraved cross on stone pillar on Inishkea North (Henry
1945, pl. XXVIII, bottom right).**

1990, 16, fig. 2), and one depicted between apposed birds in the north Italian Gospel-Book of Valerianus, now in Munich (Nordenfalk 1947, fig. 6), have similar terminals at the head and the ends of the arms. The footed *Crux Ansata* of the Coptic Glazier Codex, *c*. AD 400, in which coloured ribbon interlace appears as an integral element of illumination, also has similar spiral terminals, which are recognised by Bober (1967, 40–42, fig. 1) as typical of the period and characteristic of decorative pen-work in early manuscripts of Egyptian origin. This yoke with spiral ends is seen in developed form on the upper end of the cross-slab erected on Station 10 at Caher Island, a little to the south of the Inishkea islands (Herity 1995a, 120, fig. 30). While the Inishkea slab could be interpreted as influenced by pagan Celtic yoked designs, it is more likely, given the fact that it is footed, that the whole design, including the yokes, is derived from a cross model very like that depicted on the Baltimore medallion, in the Glazier Codex and in the Gospel-Book of Valerianus.

There is archaeological evidence of not inconsiderable trade in materials imported directly from the north-east Mediterranean to Ireland; travellers and material culture from there probably came to Ireland with the currents generated by this trade at a date relatively early in our Christian period. Wine and oil amphorae of Type Bii from Cilicia and from Antioch in ancient Syria—which, along with Jerusalem and Alexandria, was one of the three Patriarchates of the earliest Christian Church in the east Mediterranean—and Phocaean tableware of Type Ai dated between 475 and 550 from the adjacent area of modern Turkey have been found together at ecclesiastical sites and as a new feature at long-established royal and trading centres in south-west Britain and Ireland (Thomas 1959; 1981; Fulford 1989). Ralegh Radford (1956, pl. VI, A, bottom right) records crosses, one with expanded terminals like those of the *Cathach*, stamped on the inner surface of pottery dishes of Class Ai from the early monastery at Tintagel in Cornwall. These imported dishes may have had their place in Christian ritual as patens used in the Mass. One way in which east Mediterranean cross-forms like those of the *Cathach* found their way about 500 to milieux in Ireland in which manuscripts were commonly written and art in other media produced is thus documented.

Manuscript comparanda for hands, texts and decorated initials in the *Cathach*

B. Schauman (1978) recognised two Irish hands among the four hands represented in manuscript S 45 sup. of the Ambrosian Library in Milan, a copy of Jerome's *Commentaria in Isaiam* (Commentary on the Book of Isaiah), a palimpsest whose primary script is a copy of the Gothic Bible translated by Ulfila, an Arian bishop. The manuscript bears the ex-libris of Atalanus, second abbot of Bobbio, until *c.* 625, and successor of that Italian monastery's founder, Columbanus. Schauman describes it as the earliest dated manuscript from Bobbio; these two Irish hands are thus the earliest datable samples of Irish script yet known. She compares the alphabet of her Irish Hand C with that of the *Cathach*, noting that both have the diminuendo feature, that the *ductus* of the letters is very similar and that both have wedge-shaped serifs. While both use variant forms of certain letters, these variants are used in different proportions. Schauman assesses the 'formality' of Hand C and the *Cathach* hand, describing formality as a measurement of the degree of letter contiguity in a hand: where all letters are contiguous, the hand is extremely informal, where all are separated, the hand is extremely formal. Of the two hands, the *Cathach* is the 'informal' one, with a script whose sources may have been cursive. In it she recognises 'the evolution of a decorous, stately Irish script…by the steadying of the characteristics of less stately scripts with which early Irish scribes must have been familiar' (Schauman 1978, 13). Hand C may illustrate a more advanced stage in this evolution; it and Schauman's other Irish Hand D are written in a more formal script than the *Cathach* and may claim a later date than it.

Schauman also considered the possibility that the differences between these hands derive from the separate scribal traditions of Iona and its *paruchia*, to which the *Cathach* belongs, and of Bangor, to which Columbanus belonged. The two Irish hands of this Bobbio manuscript (S 45 sup.) may therefore belong to a scribal tradition practised at Bangor before 590, when Columbanus left there on the *peregrinatio* that ended with his death at Bobbio in 615. If the *Cathach* can be considered earlier than the Bobbio manuscript, then we may be inclined to give more weight than before to the possibility that it belongs to the sixth century.

In an article in the *Gazette des Beaux-Arts*, Henry (1950) notes the characteristic deformation in Celtic style of the initials in the *Cathach* and a number of Bobbio manuscripts, principally the Orosius (Ambr. D 23 sup.) and the Commentary on the Book of Isaiah by Jerome (Ambr. S 45 sup.); she also notes the incorporation of Celtic motifs in these initials. The dot-contouring of the initials, as in the early sixth-century Vienna *Dioskorides*, together with the binding in quinions and the carpet page of D 23 sup., Henry ascribes to a Coptic origin; she compares the design of the carpet page of D 23 sup. with Coptic book covers now in New York and Vienna. The simplified fish found in the *Cathach* and incorporated as a double motif in an initial *N* in MS S 45 sup. she finds in Italian manuscripts of the fifth, sixth and seventh centuries as well as in Merovingian manuscripts. She quotes Lowe (CLA², 20, 41) as noting the Irish *G* of the *Cathach* as archaic and stating that the Irish calligraphic tradition at Bangor dates to 590, when Columbanus left Bangor, or earlier. Finally, she notes that in a poem on the rule of Bangor in the seventh century Antiphonary of Bangor (MS Ambr. C 5 inf.) there is a reference to *vinea vera / ex Aegypto transducta*, possibly an oblique reference to influences from the Coptic world (Henry 1950, 9, 14, 16–18, 20, 25, 30; 1965, 64–5).

In her recent edition of the text of Orosius's world history, M.-P. Arnaud-Lindet (1990) has designated the common ancestors of all existing manuscripts as α, β and γ, representing text-types of her Classes I, II and III respectively. The immediate exemplar of manuscripts F and H of Class I (α) may have been an Irish codex from Columbanus's Luxeuil, founded before 600. The earliest extant representative of Class II is B (Milan, Ambr. D 23 sup., from Bobbio), written in insular script like that of the *Cathach* and dating from the first half of the seventh century. It is a copy of an insular exemplar β' and was taken to Bobbio from Ireland either in or shortly after the lifetime of Columbanus (died 615). Manuscripts M′ (Munich Clm. 29022, an eighth-century north Italian fragment), Q (Vat. Reg. lat. 296, written in the ninth century) and Δ (an abridgement of Orosius, probably written at Lorsch in the early ninth century) also descend from β'. Both α' and β', direct descendants of the archetypes of Classes I and II, are therefore associated with the Continental mission of Columbanus and thus derive, in one way or another, from the mother house, Bangor. The poor text in L (Florence, Bibl.

Laurentiana, Plut. 65, written in the sixth century and possibly connected with Ravenna), which is referred to above (Nordenfalk 1947), is a copy that branched off the main line of the archetype Class III (γ) and has left no descendants (Arnaud-Lindet 1990, lxxx-xc).

The *Cathach* was produced in an artistic milieu that was predominantly Irish La Tène in character. While the initials themselves and their filler motifs come from the Mediterranean, the ornamental early Christian motifs incorporated in them have a distinctive character: cross-forms, atrophied fishes and beasts and dot-contouring of the initials. Dot-contouring points to a source in Coptic contexts; the binding of manuscripts in quinions suggests an oriental source (CLA[1], vii). The cross-forms and their elaboration suggest a source in the east Mediterranean, from where distinctive pottery came to Ireland between 475 and 550. These distinctive forms are found together with marigolds on early metal ornaments and on stone carvings in early foundations throughout Ireland, from the non-Patrician province of the south-west as far north as County Down. Tradition ascribes this psalter to Colum Cille; palaeography (CLA[2], 41) and art allow the manuscript to be dated before 600. It is perhaps significant that Columbanus of Bangor and Bobbio had written an essay or treatise on the Psalms 'in elegant language' before 590, while he was still in Ireland, a copy of which was apparently taken to the continent (McNamara 1973, 222, 251–3).

Bible translations, Latin and Greek: the background to the *Cathach*

According to early tradition, the first translation of the Hebrew Pentateuch, or Law of Moses, was carried out at the behest of Pharaoh Ptolemy II Philadelphus (285–247 BC) and was into Greek. The Letter of Aristeas says that Ptolemy, at the suggestion of his librarian, dispatched an embassy to the high-priest Eleazar at Jerusalem, requesting him to send six elders from each of the twelve tribes of Israel to Alexandria, each bringing a scroll of the Law with him. Later tradition reduced this number from seventy-two to seventy, hence Septuagint (LXX). According to tradition, they completed their translations in seventy-two days. In another version, the translation was done during the reign of Ptolemy

Philometer (182–146 BC), probably with a view to encouraging the use of Greek among the Jews in his kingdom. The Septuagint is therefore the Alexandrian Greek version of the Old Testament, and the term, originally applied to the Greek translation of the Pentateuch, was later given to the entire translation. It appears that the earliest body of Greek translations was completed before 132 BC.

The Septuagint does not survive in its complete or pure form, and the existing Greek texts of some books or parts of books have been supplemented from other Greek versions. The first of these versions is by Aquila, a gentile who converted to Christianity and later to Judaism. He worked in the reign of the emperor Hadrian (AD 117–38), to whom he was related. His is a literal translation from the original Hebrew, even to the point of breaking with Greek idiom and syntax; this was well received by the Palestinian Jews, who had not approved of the Septuagint translation. The second version is by Theodotion, also a convert to Judaism, who wrote at the end of the second century AD. He revised the Septuagint against the standard Hebrew text that existed at the time and thus omitted material that had been added from other sources (for example to the Book of Daniel, the Greek text of which is longer than the Hebrew) and added material that had been omitted in the Septuagint translation, for example from the Book of Job. A third version was prepared by Symmachus (second century AD) after Theodotion. There exist fragments of three other anonymous translations, which were used by Origen (c. 185–254), mainly in his edition of the Psalms.

Origen, an Alexandrian Christian, endeavoured to restore the pure text of the Hebrew Old Testament, setting forth the text in six parallel columns—the Old Testament in Hebrew characters, the Hebrew text in Greek transcription, and the four Greek translations (the Septuagint and the three versions by Aquila, Theodotion and Symmachus). From its six-column layout it is known as the Hexapla. Origen recognised that the Greek contained clauses that were not in the Hebrew and omitted passages, some of them several chapters long, that the Hebrew contained. He edited the Greek Septuagint to conform with the Hebrew, correcting corruptions in the Septuagint that had been introduced from other manuscripts or other translations. To indicate where words or lines were missing in the Hebrew but present in the Greek he borrowed from Alexandrian philology the obelus (– or ÷); where words were wanting in the Septuagint but present in the Hebrew, he used the asterisk (*). These critical marks were later adopted by Jerome (347/8–420) for his revisions and translations from the Septuagint. Later writers, including Jerome, thought that Origen had restored the Septuagint, which had become the Greek text *par excellence* of the Church, to its pure form, and the text of the fifth column, the Hexaplaric Septuagint, was thereafter separately published. This formed the basis of Jerome's early revisions.

When Christianity spread into parts where Greek was not the common language, such as North Africa, Gaul and Italy, Latin translations were made of the Gospels and other parts of the New Testament, and, in particular, of the Psalms, which had become an integral part of the liturgy of the Church, as they were of the Jewish liturgy. Many such translations or part-translations proliferated, not all of them accurate, the text undergoing rapid and extensive development and differentiation. The Old Latin versions of the Old Testament, known as the *Vetus Latina*, survive only in fragments; almost all of the New Testament versions, because they were more prolific and more commonly used, survive. The African Church had a distinctive version of its own, known as the *Afra*, and Europe another, known as the *Itala*, of which there are several sub-forms. Eventually, so many versions existed that the situation became unmanageable and Jerome, exceptional in his time in having a knowledge of both Greek and Hebrew, was commissioned by Pope Damasus in 382 to prepare new and standard translations.

The first, published in 383, was a revision of good Latin texts of the four Gospels against a text of the Greek. Jerome states in his introduction that he made changes in the Latin only when the sense demanded it: the Gospel of Matthew was most heavily revised, that of John least. Jerome continued with further translations of groups of Old Testament books until 389, adding dedicatory epistles and historical and textual prefaces, only part of which survive. The Book of Psalms was revised twice: the first revision against the Old Latin is known as the *Romanum* (*c.* 384); the second, a more complete revision of the Old Latin against the Greek, based on the Hexapla, is known as the *Gallicanum* (*c.* 387). Both the preface and text of the *Gallicanum* survive intact (though not all of the asterisks and obeli as originally inserted by Jerome). In this Vulgate translation Jerome used the critical marks adopted by Origen, the asterisk denoting the parts of the Hebrew text omitted in the Greek of the Septuagint and the obelus marking those parts of the Septuagint not found in the Hebrew. In the preface to his correction (*Psalterium Romae dudum positus*), he asked future copyists to reproduce these critical signs along with the text itself. Jerome later abandoned the revision project in favour of a fresh translation of the Old Testament from the Hebrew, a restoration of the *Hebraica veritas*, where it still existed, and of the Aramaic where it did not (e.g. Books of Tobias and Judith). He began this translation project in 389 and continued until 405. His translation of the Psalms from the original Hebrew into Latin is known as the *Hebraicum*.

Jerome's translations were quickly corrupted by Old Latin readings where these were preferred, as they frequently were for centuries to come, so that his text of the Vulgate cannot now be recovered in its pure form. It seems clear from the evidence of the *Cathach* that the early Irish Church possessed the Psalms in both the Vulgate (*Gallicanum*) and *Hebraicum* texts.

The use of asterisk and obelus in the *Cathach*

As discussed in relation to other versions of the psalter above (pp 40–41), an asterisk indicates a passage or word in the Hebrew that is missing from the Greek, an obelus a passage or word missing from the Hebrew but found in the Greek. In the *Cathach*, the obeli can be palaeographically distinguished from the faint 'division signs' that were added in at the end of certain lines to mark verse or part-verse divisions (corresponding with the *stichoi* of the Greek text). The obeli are larger than the division signs, are in the same ink as the main text and were copied at the same time as it.

There are twenty-five uses of the obelus (Fig. 18) in the *Cathach*, indicating omissions from the Hebrew. Four of these (at Psalms 89:17b; 91:10a; 94:9c; 97:5) are placed before words that are in Jerome's *Hebraicum* but are missing from the Irish family of this translation, represented in the manuscript group AKI (comprising the Codex **A**miatinus, Florence, dated *ante* 716; **K**arlsruhe Cod. Aug. XXXVIII, ninth century; and the Psalter of

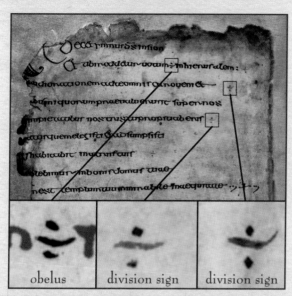

obelus   division sign   division sign

Fig. 18—Fol. 25v of *Cathach*, showing obelus and division signs.

St Ouen (siglum **I**), tenth century, the oldest and purest text of the three) and others. They therefore represent not Jerome's original *Hebraicum* but a revision of the *Gallicanum* against the Irish *Hebraicum*, indicating words missing from or altered in the (Irish) *Hebraicum* but present in the *Gallicanum*. In two places, the obeli are misplaced, at Psalm 84:12a, where ÷ *et veritas* is not omitted in either the Hebrew, Greek or Latin, and at Psalm 104:44a, *in laetitia ÷ et dedit illis*, where the obelus should have been placed before the *et* at the beginning of the verse (÷ *et electos suos in laetitia...*), where there is an omission in the *Hebraicum*. The omission of ÷ *et in bracchio* (Psalm 88:11b) represents a variant of the Gallican Vulgate found in the *Cathach* and in the Psalter of St Ouen (MS Rouen, Bibl. Mun. 24). The rest of the obeli represent omissions from the established *Hebraicum*. The presence of corrections from the Irish family of the *Hebraicum* can be explained in two ways: (i) the Irish schools had a text of Jerome's *Hebraicum* peculiar to themselves at some indeterminate time before the *Cathach* was written; (ii) they had compared the text of the *Gallicanum* against that of the *Hebraicum* in order to present in a single text the results of both of Jerome's critical translations. This collation was present in the exemplar of the *Cathach* also; the exemplar may even have been a double psalter, with the *Gallicanum* and *Hebraicum* on alternate pages, of which the *Cathach* scribe copied only the *Gallicanum*. This indicates that a certain amount of early critical-textual work on the psalter was being done in the Irish schools, in McNamara's (1973, 267) opinion 'at a very early date in the sixth century at the latest'. Just how much was done, and what the methodology of these sixth-century scholars was, remain to be explored. Certainly the Irish knew the purpose of these critical signs, apart from merely copying them from their sources: this is evident from, among other sources, the Treatise on the Psalter in Old Irish (thought to be eighth century) and from the letter of the anonymous Irishman in Milan on the emendation of the Latin psalter against the Greek (ninth century) (McNamara 1973, 229–30, 235–7). There is therefore method and purpose behind the use of these signs in the *Cathach*.

There are twenty-two uses of the asterisk (Fig. 19) in the *Cathach*. One (Psalm 53:3b) was written by the scribe over an erasure, and three were entered as editorial restorations in the now mutilated fragment (Psalms 58:6a; 73:15b; 92:3c). Nine of the twenty-two asterisks correspond to Jerome's original Gallican text. Five further asterisks occur in places where there are words in the Hebrew that are not in the Greek; these are correctly under asterisk even though they are absent in the text of Jerome's *Gallicanum* as we have it. One of the five, at Psalm 34:20b, may have had an asterisk in Jerome's original *Gallicanum*; the remaining four (Psalms 53:5c; 70:8a; 77:21a; 88:45b) represent additions in the Irish *Gallicanum*. With the exception of Psalm 77:21a, all of these variants also have Greek, Syriac and/or Old Latin support. A further asterisk at Psalm 85:12a represents an omission in some manuscripts of one branch of the Greek text.

The remaining seven asterisks are placed against passages that are in the Greek. Five of them are placed against words present in all texts of the psalter—the Hebrew, the Greek, the Old Latin and the *Gallicanum*. Two of them can readily be explained: the omission of *et* in Psalm 49:7 (*Israhel ∗ et*) may be a misplacement of the asterisk before the word preceding *Israhel, tibi*, which is omitted in several Greek and Latin sources. Similarly, in Psalm 103:7 *tonitrui ∗ tui* is an error by the scribe, since *tui* is an omission from three Irish manuscripts of the *Hebraicum* (group RAK—R being the eighth-century Codex Reginensis; A and K as above) and should therefore be marked with an obelus. The other five (Psalms 34:15a; 53:3b; 58:6a; 65:7a; 85:4b) do not at present permit any explanation, unless they are simply errors.

Our present 'accepted' text of the Septuagint Greek psalter (Rahlfs 1979) is a reconstruction from the extant witnesses: there is no reason to assume that the Greek from which the text of the *Cathach* is ultimately derived was identical with it, and the possibility that the ancestral text of the *Cathach* was not simply a text of the 'pure' *Gallicanum* but a particular text of the Greek against which the *Gallicanum* was compared should be examined. There are also other possible explanations for these anomalies in the use of asterisk and obelus, e.g. copying errors or misplacements resulting from the simultaneous collation of two (or even more) versions of the Latin psalter.

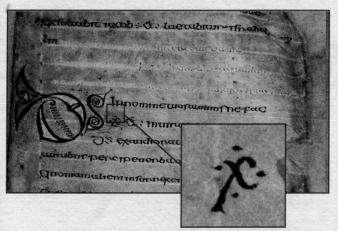

Fig. 19—Fol. 19r of *Cathach*, showing rubric and asterisk.

The rubrics in the *Cathach* and what they contain

The rubrics, or headings (see illustration above), were added by the *prima manus* in orange ink above the text of each psalm proper in a more uncial hand after the main text was written. In some cases the scribe left insufficient room, so that a word or phrase occasionally had to be disposed in the margins. This technique of adding rubricated headings in spaces left for them in the main text can also be found in Egyptian (Coptic) illumination.

They were clearly not added to the *Cathach* as an *aide memoire*, since the ancients learned the psalter by heart, and psalmody was not done with a book (Dyer 1989; Woolfenden 1993). The *Cathach* was probably kept for private reading and study or as a special possession. We do not know if it was used for communal monastic service.

Each psalm in the *Cathach* has a tripartite heading giving, where they have been copied or are fully preserved, (i) a heading proper (verse 1 of each psalm, from the Greek text, the Septuagint), (ii) what has been taken by Lawlor, Salmon and others as some liturgical instruction (e.g. Psalm 47: *legendus ad Apocalipsim Iohannis*) but is more probably a devotional directive (Dyer 1989, 69–70), and (iii) an interpretative heading or *titulus*. Several such series of headings, deriving from different Fathers, were identified and edited by Dom Pierre Salmon (Salmon 1959; 1962). The series of *tituli* in the *Cathach* is the oldest, and the *Cathach*, being the second oldest Latin psalter now in existence, is also the earliest representative of that series, designated Series I. Only the devotional/liturgical headings, where they are present, and the *tituli* proper were edited by Dom Salmon (Salmon 1959, 48–74). He identified six series: with the exception of Series I, they can all be quite readily dated and their source(s) identified. Series IV derives from the psalm commentary of Eusebius of Caesarea (*c*. 265–339) and is found in the famous Greek Codex Alexandrinus (fifth century); it survives in an Old Latin translation that first appears in Carolingian psalters of the eighth to ninth century. Series III derives from the homilies of Origen of Alexandria (*c*. 185–254) on the psalms in the translation of Jerome. Series V and II are of fourth- and fifth-century derivation respectively. The most recent series is VI, which derives from Cassiodorus (*c*. 485–580), later adapted by Bede (673–735). These series were thus composed between the end of the third and the end of the sixth century. The authors of the Series IV and VI, Eusebius and Cassiodorus, are known. Although we know the ultimate sources of the other series, we do not know the circumstances of their composition or early dissemination. The oldest texts are the most concise, the later series more elaborate and wordy. All the ancient psalters, Latin and Greek, contain this material, whether in the form of collective summaries or as rubrics before each individual psalm, as they appear in the *Cathach*. Their purpose, as Dom Salmon has pointed out, is to orient prayer and to facilitate interpretation, that is, to identify the speaker or *persona* of each psalm and give it a coherent interpretation.

For the Church of the martyrs and the early Fathers, the psalter was a book about Christ, and each psalm was either *vox de Christo*, *vox ecclesiae ad Christum* or *vox Christi ad Patrem*. The Christological interpretation of the psalms, i.e. the interpretation of them as referring to Christ or the events of his life, can first be found in the citations from them in the Acts of the Apostles and in the Book of Hebrews in the New Testament, e.g. the use of Psalm 16:10 in Acts 2:27, Psalm 2:7 in Hebrews 1:5 and Psalm 8:5–7 in Hebrews 2:6–8. This mode of interpretation was continued thereafter by Justin Martyr, Irenaeus, Clemens of Alexandria and most of the major Greek Fathers (Linton 1961). The Christological series found in the *Cathach* is doubly valuable, since its roots are in early Christianity and the *Cathach* is the earliest known manuscript witness to it. Its sources have not been identified, and most modern authorities are content to state that it is not possible to determine whether it is native or transmitted to Ireland. The sources are certainly not Latin, although there are tenuous connections with Tertullian and Augustine. Dom Salmon (1959, 53) has noted the close correspondence between the interpretative heading to Psalm 1, *De Joseph dicit qui corpus Christi sepelivit* (defective in the *Cathach*), and the exegesis of Tertullian as well as some similarities with the exegesis of Augustine in Psalms 48, 50, 56, 60, 86, 90 and 115. There are Christological elements in both Jerome's Shorter Commentaries on the Psalms (*Commentarioli in Psalmos*) and Augustine's great commentary, but they are quite different from the *Cathach tituli*, which do not conform to the interpretative headings given by either. It can now be shown that Dom Salmon's assertion, 'Certain elements of these series, especially of the first one, may go back to the third century' (Salmon 1962, 51), has some truth and that the *tituli* of Series I bear a striking similarity to some Greek psalm commentaries.

Although the rubrics of Series I can be separated into three parts, there is no manuscript evidence that these three elements circulated separately. Also, in the *Cathach* at least, the three headings clearly form an integrated text. Unfortunately, because of the fragmentary and poor preservation of the *Cathach*, and

partly because of scribal errors, many of these headings are
missing, corruptly or incompletely preserved or illegible.

The first element, the *titulus* of each psalm, being th
verse, was taken from the Septuagint into Jerome's c
revision against it, the *Gallicanum*. The text of the *Cathach*
differs in some respects from the *tituli* of the critical *Gallic*
in the Vatican and Stuttgart editions and agrees more closel
those of Eusebius of Caesarea and other Greek Fathers
second element, the devotional rubric (*legendus ad…*), m
some cases also derive from the same source(s) that provid
inscriptiones, or headings, and the *tituli*. For example, Euse
exegesis of Psalm 44:10–16 is suggestive of the devotional
in the *Cathach*, *Legendus ad evangelium Mathei de regina*
(cf. Matthew 11:42, Luke 11:31). Also, Eusebius's
Athanasius's exegeses of Psalm 68:1 (as well as the text
psalm itself, of course) bear a very close affinity to the *C*
titulus, *Legendus ad lectionem Jonae prophetae…vox Chris*
pateretur: the psalm is associated with a reading from the p
Jonah (probably chapter 2, Jonah's prayer of affliction
belly of the whale), and the *vox* of the psalm is that of Ch
his suffering. The *titulus* can certainly be recovered fro
exegesis of these Fathers, and the devotional link is (
suggested in some texts. Similarly, Eusebius's exegesis of
47 suggests its association with Apocalypse 21, on the vis
the New Jerusalem.

The third element is of most interest in determinir
textual antecedents of the *Cathach*. Dom Salmon (1962,
has shown that the *Cathach* series is the source from which
other witnesses to Series I derive, via its transmission to E
in the seventh century. The subsequent history of the serie
little interest in this context but has been studied in some
by Lawlor (1916, 413–35) and amplified by Salmon
51–4). The series is designated Christological, that
persona, where identified, is denoted *propheta* and the *vo*
addresses, of the psalms are in almost all cases attribu
Christ, the apostles or the Church. To give a rather in
example, Psalm 44, slightly corrupt in the *Cathach*,
Propheta pro patre de Christo et ecclesia dicit, that is, the
is to be interpreted as the words of the Father, throu
prophet, to or of Christ and the Church, specifically of the (
called from among the Gentiles.

In fact, the majority of the *tituli* bear some similarity to the exegesis of Eusebius of Caesarea (*c.* 265–339) (PG 23, 441C–1221C) and to that of Athanasius of Alexandria (295–373) (PG 27, 60C–545C), whose dependence on the exegesis of Eusebius (Rondeau 1958; Vian 1991, 16) and, to a lesser extent, on the exegesis of Gregory of Nyssa (died 394) has been demonstrated (McDonough 1962; Heine 1995). Eusebius's vast commentary is based upon the Hexaplaric text and the commentaries of his mentor, Origen of Alexandria, to which he had direct access; both commentaries survive only in fragments. Eusebius gives the historical or literal exegesis of each psalm as well as its metaphorical interpretation, with some explanation of the *voces* and *personae* of the psalm. The *Cathach tituli* refer to the sense of the psalm as a whole or to a specific verse in it and are terse to the point of obscurity. The commentaries, however, being extended exegeses of the psalms, do not always convey the substance of the *titulus* at the beginning, where one might expect to find it. Instead, this information is sometimes diffused throughout the text and at other times conveyed within the exegesis of a specific verse or phrase of the psalm. Athanasius is much more succinct in his exposition than Eusebius and is therefore easier to use as a source. Eusebius's exegesis is both Alexandrian and Antiochean, that is both allegorical and historical, although it leans toward the former. The commentary of Athanasius, the great representative of the Alexandrian school of exegesis, is distinctly allegorical.

There is no extant translation of Eusebius's commentary, although Jerome, who cannot always be relied on, states that Eusebius of Vercelli made a translation of it into Latin in the fourth century (*De uiris illustribus*, §96). There is evidence that Hilary of Poitiers (*c.* 310–367/8) was familiar with parts of Eusebius's commentary (especially Psalms 1:65 and 188) and may have translated it, although his own exegesis, especially *Tractatus super Psalmos*, mainly relies on the now very fragmentary commentaries of Origen. It is certainly possible that the text of one or other of these translations was known in the Irish schools or that an ancient Latin psalter containing headings derived from Eusebius's commentary reached Ireland. However, in the complete absence of any trace of those translations it is not possible to make definitive statements. Some of the *Cathach* series of headings may very well be the product of an indigenous

Irish tradition of psalm interpretation based on careful study of Scripture, of which there is ample evidence from the early Irish monastic schools. It is not likely that all of them are the product of native invention, independent of any outside influence or source. The links with the commentaries of Eusebius, Athanasius and Gregory are almost certainly not direct, but some connection with the Alexandrian tradition of exegesis seems quite possible given the proven patristic derivation of the other five series and in the absence of any provable dependence upon the Latin Fathers.

The sources of some of the headings remain unidentified. The *titulus* to Psalm 64, *vox ecclesiae ante baptismum paschalismatum*, is particularly unusual. The hapax or unique occurrence of the word '*paschalismatum*' is a loan translation from Greek, being a neuter Latin adjective derived from πασχαλισμός. The *titulus* may have liturgical significance (Salmon 1959, 52) or it may refer to the 'baptism' of the Church in Christ's blood, his passion. A fuller investigation of the *tituli* and their sources would greatly help our understanding of their tripartite structure (where it exists) and text. They were almost certainly transmitted together as a unit from an ancient psalter that underwent refinements and additions from native tradition.

The language of the *tituli* has a number of peculiarities that may indicate some dependence on a Greek source, especially the use of the Graecisms *exomologessem* in Psalm 43 (*ex homo legessem* in the *Cathach*) and *paschalismatum* in Psalm 64 (only a fragment of the word is visible in the *Cathach*). The peculiarities of the syntax and language deserve comment—for example, the *titulus* to Psalm 35, *Profeta cum laude opera ipsius Iudae dicit,* and the strange phraseology of Psalm 36, *...monet ad fidei firmamentum.* Salmon also noted these peculiarities but took them to be liturgical elements in the headings. The liturgical heading to Psalm 26, *Legendus ad lectionem Esaiae prophetae: ecce qui serviunt tibi bona manducabunt* (Isaiah 65:13 paraphrased from the Old Latin; defective in the *Cathach*), would lead one to suspect that the Old and New Testament readings for use or meditation in conjunction with each psalm were of the Old Latin type. There are similarities here with the bilingual Easter Vigil lections and the forty short readings from the Minor Prophets in the codex known as *Liber Commonei* (Oxford, Bodleian Library, MS Auct. F.4./32, dated 817): the Latin texts in this ancient collection have a peculiar phraseology that is indicative of their accommodation to a Greek original, and are distinctly pre-Vulgate in type (Fischer 1952; Hunt 1961; Lapidge 1983; Breen 1992).

Several examples of correspondence between the *Cathach* and the commentaries of Eusebius, Athanasius and/or Gregory have been isolated. A systematic examination of other patristic commentaries that are likely to bear some relationship to the *Cathach* series—such as those of Hesychius of Jerusalem, Didymus of Alexandria or Diodore of Tarsus—has not been made, nor has the content of every *titulus* in the *Cathach*, ending at Psalm 105, been examined. Further research would undoubtedly bring to light many more correspondences. The following are a few examples, chosen for their brevity and clarity from a longer list, as illustrations of close similarity with the commentaries of each of the three Fathers Eusebius, Athanasius and Gregory. All citations from patristic sources are given in the modern Latin translation in Migne (PG) to facilitate direct comparison with the *Cathach*. The Greek original has not been quoted, except for the purpose of illustration.

Recent researches by McNamara (1998; 1999) have indicated plausible similarities between the *Cathach* series and other Latin Psalm commentaries, including the early seventh-century *Glosa Psalmorum ex traditione Seniorum*, but they demonstrate no direct dependence either way. The source(s) from which the *Cathach* derived its *tituli* series can certainly be placed well within the sixth century, earlier than any of the comparanda adduced from later medieval Latin tradition. Suggestive verbal coincidences indicated by McNamara between the texts of the individual psalms and their headings in the *Cathach* series only show that the series was informed at source by the exegesis of the psalms, which is no more than what one would expect. It does not prove that this series, alone of the six, was *sui generis*. The question of its dependence upon a Greek source therefore remains a plausible hypothesis.

The sources of the *tituli* in the *Cathach*

In the following, *Cathach* headings are represented in bold typeface (with spelling following Lawlor's transcription); underlining represents the author's highlighting of similarities between the *Cathach* headings and the commentaries of the Fathers; direct quotations from the Bible cited by the Fathers in their commentaries are placed between quotation marks. The figures in parentheses immediately preceding quotations from commentaries of Athanasius, Eusebius or Gregory refer to the volume and column numbers in Migne (PG); volume and column numbers are separated by a semicolon.

(1) Psalm 32:1—**Psalmus Dauid. profeta cum laude dei populum hortatur**
Athanasius, *Expositio in Psalmos*, at Psalm 32: 1 (PG 27; 163/4)—<u>In presenti docet eos qui jam in Christum crediderunt laudare Dominum suum</u>

The *Cathach* heading means 'the prophet exhorts the people with [or to] the praise of God', and Athanasius interprets it similarly.[9]

(2) Psalm 34:1—**Huic Dauid. uox Christi in passione de Iudaeis dicit**
Athanasius, *Expositio in Psalmos*, at Psalm 34:1 (PG 27; 169/70)—<u>Inducitur item persona Christi ea ennarantis quae sibi tempore Passionis a Iudaeis illata sunt mala</u>

The psalm begins 'Judge thou O Lord them that wrong me'. The *Cathach titulus* and Athanasius are in complete agreement: the voice of Christ in his Passion speaks of the wrongs committed against him by the Jews.

(3) Psalm 35:1—**profeta cum laude opera ipsius Iudae dicit**
This heading, inserted by Lawlor from manuscripts ABRS (cf. Lawlor 1916, 242–3, for key to manuscripts) is no longer present in the *Cathach*; its absence is noted in Salmon's apparatus

---

[9] The translations of *Cathach* headings in this booklet are Aidan Breen's. Readers should note that the headings in the English version of the psalms on the CD-ROM do not necessarily match those in the *Cathach*; in particular, the English version (Challoner's edition of the Douay-Rheims translation) does not always include details of the *persona* or *voces* of the respective psalms.

criticus (Salmon 1959, 59). The heading, despite the preponderance of MS witnesses to it, may be somewhat corrupt. Two MSS (Vat. lat. 84 and Vat. lat. 12985) add a following phrase, construing the psalm as a prophetic accusation against the Jewish people (*ejusque est accusatio de populo judaico*; cf. Series II). Athanasius's exegesis is very similar to both of these:

Athanasius, *Expositio in Psalmos,* at Psalm 35:1 (PG 27; 173/6)—Superbiae Judaici populi accusationem continet hic Psalmus...atque justa Dei judicia decantat, quod orbem condiderit. Ad haec etiam gratiarum actionem Patri offert pro beneficiis per Jesum collatis... 'Iniquitatem meditatus est in cubiculo suo...' (Psalm 35:5) Vigiles et insomnes noctes eorum qui Christo insidias parabant significat... Judaei enim mysterium per leges et prophetas edocti exciderunt, gentes vero...assumptae sunt...

The correct translation of the Latin might be: 'the prophet speaks with praise of His [i.e. God's] works to Juda [i.e. the Jewish people, or Judas the traitor].'

(4) Psalm 39:1—**patientia populi est**

Athanasius, *Expositio in Psalmos,* Psalm 39:2 (PG 27; 189/90)—Refertur canticum ex persona novi populi de lacu miseriae reducti... Expectans expectavi Dominum, et intendit mihi (Psalm 39:2). Simile huic: 'In patientia vestra possidebitis animas vestras' (Luke 21:19).

Athanasius cites the text 'in your patience shall you possess your souls' as a proof of the meaning of the psalm; the persona is that of the new people of the Word (ἐκ προσώπου τοῦ νέου λαοῦ).

(5) Psalm 43:1—**hic ex homo legessem[10] legendus ad epistolam Pauli ad Romanos. profeta ad dominum de operibus eius paenitentiam gerens pro populo Iudaico**

Eusebius, *Commentarii in Psalmos*, at Psalm 43 (PG 23; 383/6)—nimirum de ruina Judaici populi, ex prophetarum

---

[10] for ex homo legessem *read* exomolegesim.

persona a filiis Core prolatae... In superioribus itaque lacryma-bantur, doloremque suum Deo renuntiabant; in presenti vero ipsas calamitates ennarant... 'Deum celebrabimus tota die, et nomini tuo confitebimur in aeternum' (Psalm 43:9). Confessionem (ἐξομολόγησιν) porro pro gratiarum actione usurpare Scripturae solent... Sed haec quidem ex persona chori prophetici dicta sunt. Quae vero deinde feruntur iidem rursus, multitudinis casus sibi ascribentes, ennarant... Quoniam multitudo totius populi Judaici, in omni impietatis et improbitatis genere volutata, non aliena erat a corpore prophetarum, populi aerumnas sibi proprias attribuentes...Haec tam multa chorus propheticus in sua ad Deum supplicatione, calamitates populi ascribens sibi, prosecutus est.

Athanasius, *Expositio in Psalmos,* Psalm 43:18 (PG 27; 205/6)—'haec omnia venerunt...' (Psalm 43:18) Jam diximus prophetas esse qui ex populi persona supplicationes offerunt, quasi propria sibi reputantes mala ipsi peccatorum causa obvenientia.

The words of the psalm are those of the prophet(s) to God, attributing to themselves the tribulations and calamities which have befallen the Jewish people.

(6) Psalm 44:1—**legendus ad euangelium Mathei de regina austri. profeta ad** [Salmon reads **pro**] **patre de Christo et ecclesia dicit**

Eusebius, *Commentarii in Psalmos,* at Psalm 68 (PG 23; 721/2)—Quadragesimus itaque quartus de Dilecto prophetiam, atque gentium Ecclesiae a pejoribus ad meliora immutationem, complectitur...

and again at Psalm 44 (PG 23; 391/394)—ut intelligamus totam sermonis seriem canticum pro Dilecto complecti; aut... 'Canticum in Dilectum' (Psalm 44:1)... Dilectum autem illum esse Unigenitum Dei Filium... 'Dominus dabit Verbum evangelizantibus virtute multa. Rex virtutum Dilecti' (Psalm 67:12–13); ubi aperte ac speciatim Dominus Deus universorum memoratur (Σαφῶς δὲ κανταῦθα ἰδίως μνημονευομένου Κυρίου τοῦ Θεοῦ τῶν ὅλων); ac rursum speciatim Dilectus, ac demum tertio ordine, evangelizantes Dilectum, quibus ab ipso Deo Verbum dari...Hic adjiciatur ad sermonem totum obsignandum, salutare Evangelium paterna voce Dilectum apud homines clamore edito commonstrasse: 'Hic est Filius meus dilectus, in quo mihi complacui' (Matthew 17:5). Tot tantisque de Dilecto prolatis, plane demum ac sine contradictione fuerit haec prophetia in titulo sic enuntiata: 'Canticum pro Dilecto' (Psalm 44:1). Quod autem hic ipse Christus, alius ab eo, qui ipsum iniunxit Patre, in eodem Psalmo postea declaratur... Quidam arbitrati sunt ex persona Patris Psalmum sive canticum pronuntiari de Verbo... <u>Mihi porro haec ad propheticum chorum referenda videntur.</u>

Athanasius, *Expositio in Psalmos*, Psalm 44:1 (PG 27; 207/14)—Praesens canticum David offert, scilicet Christo... 'Eructavit cor meum verbum bonum' (Psalm 44:2). Hoc Pater ait de Filio: genitus namque est Deus ex Deo.

Eusebius (PG 23; 951) isolates the three elements in the *titulus* of this psalm: (i) that it is a prophecy expressed through David (cf. also Athanasius), (ii) that it is in the 'voice', or on behalf of the Father (cf. also Athanasius), and (iii) that it relates to Christ and the calling of the Church from the gentiles. The *persona* of the psalm is not God the Father but the prophet. The early Church interpreted this psalm as messianic: Psalm 44:7–8 (Sedis tua Deus in saeculum saeculi virga directionis virga regni tui. Dilexisti iustitiam et odisti iniquitatem. Proptera unxit te Deus Deus tuus oleo laetitiae prae consortibus tuis.) is taken to refer to Christ in Hebrews 1:8–9. This is also the understanding of the *Cathach* heading.

(7) Psalm 52:1—**In finem pro Melech intelligentia Dauid legendus ad euangelium Mathei. increpat Iudeos incredulos operibus negantes deum**

Gregory of Nyssa, *In inscriptiones Psalmorum*, at Psalm 52 (PG 44; 566)—'inutiles facti sunt omnes' (Psalm 52:4)... Dominus igitur propter haec 'de caelo respexit super filios hominum' (Psalm 52:2). <u>Quae verba Domini inter homines conversationem indicant, quando praeeuntes ad incredulitatem sacerdotes et Pharisaeos, et Scribas, omnes subditi secuti sunt: illi enim erant, qui blasphemis suis dentibus populum laniabant et devorabant.</u>

The Lord rebukes the unbelieving Jews, especially the priests, Pharisees and Scribes, who by their deeds deny God and with their blasphemies destroy the people.

(8) Psalm 54:1—In finem intellectus in carminibus Dauid. uox Christi aduersus magnatos Iudeorum et de Iuda traditore

Eusebius, *Commentarii in Psalmos*, Psalm 54:13–14 (PG 23; 474)—Ex quibus omnibus aestimo non posse ad Davidis personam haec referri; sed <u>prophetica</u> vi arbitror dicta esse, <u>et in uno Salvatore et Domino nostro completa, quando Judaicae gentis principes</u>, <u>Hierosolymae in unum congregati, consessum ac consilium inierunt, quomodo eum perderent</u>. ('Εξ ὧν ἀπάντων ἡγοῦμαι μὴ χώραν ἔχειν ἀναφέρεσθαι τὰ προκείμενα ἐπὶ τὸ τοῦ Δαυιδ πρόσωπον· προφητικῇ δέ οἷμαι δυνάμει λελέχθαι αὐτά, καὶ ἐπὶ μόνον τὸν Σωτῆρα καὶ Κύριον ἡμῶν συνίστασθαι πεπληρωμένα, ὅτε, κατὰ τὸ αὐτὸ συναχθέντες οἱ τοῦ Ἰουδαίων ἔθνους ἄρχοντες ἐπὶ τῆς Ἱερουσαλὴμ, συνέδριον ἐποιήσαντο καὶ σκέψιν ὅπως αὐτὸν ἀπολέσωσιν· ἐν ᾧ οἱ μὲν θάνατον αὐτοῦ κατεψηφίσαντο)...<u>Aperte porro Evangelii scriptura prophetiam asserit, haec de proditore Juda accipiens</u>, (ἐπὶ τὸν προδότην Ἰούδαν ἐκλαβοῦσα τὸ) '<u>Si inimicus meus maledixisset mihi, sustinuissem utique</u>…' (Psalm 54:13)

The words of the Psalm inveigh against the great ones of the Jewish people when they conspired to do away with Christ, and against Judas the traitor.

(9) Psalm 57:1—In finem ne disperdas Dauid. In tituli inscriptione profeta denioribus [*lege*: de senioribus] Iudaeorum dicit.

Eusebius, *Commentarii in Psalmos*, at Psalm 57:7 (PG 23. 531/2)—Animadvertendum autem est, num <u>prophetia isthaec, quae tota cohaeret et una serie jungitur cum praecedentibus. finem describat eorum, qui prophetias de Christo meditantur. justitiam ore loquuntur, et venientem ipsum receperunt; neque tamen vocem eius audierunt qua clamabat ipsis haec dicens: 'Qui habet aures audiendi audiat' (Mt. 11:5): qui sese serpenti similes effecerunt, et aures sibi pararunt 'sicut aspides surdae et</u>

obturantis aures suas' (Psalm 57:5). Ii vero ipsi dentes suos molasque suas blasphemis in Salvatorem nostrum dictis exacuerunt ...(Οἱ δὲ αὐτοὶ καὶ τοῦ' ὀδόντας αὐτῶν καὶ τας μύλας διὰ τῶν κατὰ τοῦ Σωτῆρος ἡμῶν βλασφημιῶν ἠκόνησαν)...Possunt item haec dici de omnibus qui athea dogmata, et impias falsasque sententias in atheis heresibus consarcinarunt, atque de iis qui sapientiam huius saeculi profitentur, qui linguas suas contra salutarem doctrinam exacuerunt.

Eusebius implicitly equates those who blaspheme the Lord with the Elders of Israel.

(10) Ps 58:1—vox Christi de Iudeis ad patrem

Eusebius, *Commentarii in Psalmos*, at Psalm 58 (PG 23; 537/8C)—Exsurge in occursum meum, et vide. Deinde vero, tanta usus fiducia, <u>a prophetico spiritu illustratur, ac ediscit futurum tempus, quo ipse Christus Dei vexationibus et insidiis Judaici populi impetetur, ac servator et inspector universarum gentium erit</u>.

(φωτίζεται ὑπό τοῦ προφητικοῦ πνεύματος, καὶ διδάσκεται, ὡς ἄρα ἔσται τις καιρὸς ἐν ᾧ καὶ ὁ Χριστὸς τοῦ θεοῦ διωχθήσεται, καὶ ἐπιδουλευθήσεται ὑπὸ τοῦ Ἰουδαίων ἔθνους, σωτήρ τε καὶ ἐπίσκοπος τῶν ἐθνῶν ἁπάντων γενήσεται)

(11) Psalm 68:1—legendus ad lectionem Ionae profetae et ad euangelium Iohannis. vox Christi cum pateretur

Athanasius, *Expositio in Psalmos*, Psalm 68:15–16 (PG 27; 305/6)—<u>Continet psalmus precationem Salvatoris, ex persona humanitatis oblatam, et narrat quae causae fuerint quod ei mortem crucis obtulerint. Insuper ipsam passionem clare narrat</u>... 'Libera me ab iis qui oderunt me et de profundis aquarum' et 'Non me demergat tempestas aquae' (Psalm 53:15–16).

Eusebius, *Commentarii in Psalmos*, at Psalm 68 (PG 23, 723/4)—<u>Quare dixeris prophetiam esse ex persona Servatoris nostri enarrantis ea quae sibi postea contigerunt; praedictionemque eorum quae Judaeis post tantos ausus illata sunt</u>. Orditur itaque Servator orationem emittens ad Patrem his verbis:

'Salvum me fac, Deus, quoniam intraverunt aquae usque ad animam meam' (Psalm 68:2) .... Ipse igitur quem non alium esse quam Dei Verbum superius demonstravimus, orationem effundit ad Patrem, hominis quem assumpsit cruciatus sibi proprios reputans, quare ait: 'Salvum me fac, Deus, quoniam intraverunt aquae usque ad animam meam. Infixus sum in limo profundi, et non est substantia. Veni in altitudinem maris, et tempestas demersit me' (Psalm 68:2–3).

Both exegeses interpret the Psalm as the words of Christ on his passion, spoken prophetically through David. The association with the story of Jonah is implicit from the reference to drowning in the watery depths.

Some provisional conclusions can be drawn from the above examples:

1. The series of *tituli* exemplified in the *Cathach* bears a strong relation to the psalm exegesis of some of the Greek Fathers, especially Eusebius of Caesarea, Athanasius and probably— but to a lesser extent—Gregory of Nyssa. Direct dependence on any one of these commentaries cannot be sustained, for two reasons. Firstly, because (to my knowledge) we have no Greek series of *tituli* to compare directly with the *Cathach* or other cognate Latin MS witnesses, and so we lack comparative textual evidence on which to base a firmer hypothesis. Secondly, several of the *Cathach* headings have not yet been traced, not even the source of Psalm 64, with its rare Greek word *paschalismos*. Since there is nothing comparable in the Greek sources so far examined for a number of the *tituli*, clearly not all the sources or, more precisely, all the congeners of the series have been traced. The imperfections in our extant manuscript sources must also be taken into account. With the exception of Gregory's *De titulis Psalmorum*, of which a critical edition has recently been published (Heine 1995), the enormous commentaries of Eusebius, Athanasius and others are still only available in imperfect early editions, reprinted in PG (Migne). The headings in the *Cathach* were copied, sometimes inaccurately, from an Irish exemplar, and it is quite evident that this exemplar had in turn taken them from its exemplar. In each case, therefore, we are working at several removes from the

original documents; we must therefore take care not to make hasty inferences.

2. If the parallels with the Greek texts so far scrutinised are merely a coincidence in interpretative tradition, one must nonetheless explain the evident Graecisms of syntax and vocabulary in the *tituli* in some other way and dismiss as purely coincidental the close similarities in thought and even vocabulary between the *Cathach* series and the Greek texts. This is not to dismiss or minimise the evidence that the liturgical rubrics and *tituli* might be the product of a living tradition of exegesis in early medieval Ireland. The sources, Latin and Greek, of the other series of *tituli* have been identified. No doubt such series were later modified and added to (and many are confused with each other in the manuscripts), but they were not manufactured *ex nihilo*, and they clearly belong to an ancient and continuous Christian tradition of giving specificChristological interpretations to many of the psalms.

3. The full three-part headings in the *Cathach* are almost certainly the product of a tradition of exegesis and not the work of an isolated scholar. Whether that tradition is entirely indigenous or relied upon imported material—the latter being far more probable at this very early period—cannot be established. It does seem likely, however, that the series was transmitted to the Western Church intact, probably in an ancient psalter, and thence to Ireland at a very early date, in the fifth or early sixth century. The tradition of exegesis is also witnessed in later Irish exegetical material on the psalms. If the psalms of this series were composed in Ireland, it is hard to believe that a school of Irish biblical scholars chanced quite coincidentally upon interpretative headings so similar, for the entire range of the psalms, to those in the sources that we have examined. If the original source(s) of the series is/are Greek, this merely adds to the growing body of evidence in support of the transmission of liturgical and other materials of Greek origin (like bodies of *onomastica sacra* and possibly a number of patristic texts) to Ireland from diverse locations. These materials were then preserved in Latin form in the host country.

Conclusions

Elements of the both the ornament and the codicology of the *Cathach* point to influence from early Christian sources in the eastern Mediterranean. Specifically, the cross-forms indicate influence from the non-Latin provinces of the late Roman Empire in that part of the Mediterranean within the late fifth and early sixth centuries. Examination of the codicology suggests that these artistic influences are mirrored in the distinctive traces of Greek derivation in the verse structure and in other features revealed by the exegesis of the psalm *tituli*, which, though now imperfectly preserved within the manuscript, appear to derive ultimately from the Alexandrian Church. The authors, arguing from very different sets of material, reinforce the opinions of Lowe, Schauman and others that there is nothing in the form or the detailed structure of the text of the *Cathach* that would argue against a date of origin before 600.

It is hoped that further research on this important Irish manuscript, now made available by computer technology for scrutiny by scholars in all relevant disciplines throughout the world, will continue to clarify and enhance our understanding and appreciation of its textual and cultural context.

References

Abbreviated references

AFM   O'Donovan, J. (ed.) 1856 *Annála Ríoghachta Éireann. Annals of the Kingdom of Ireland, by the Four Masters, from the earliest period to the year 1616* (2nd edn). Dublin. Hodges, Smith and Co.

AI   Mac Airt, S. (ed.) 1951 *The Annals of Inisfallen.* Dublin. Dublin Institute for Advanced Studies.

AU   Mac Airt, S. and Mac Niocaill, G. (eds) 1983 *The Annals of Ulster (to AD 1131).* Dublin. Dublin Institute for Advanced Studies.

AT   Stokes, W. (ed.) 1895–7 The Annals of Tigernach. *Revue Celtique* **16**, 374–419; **17**, 6–33, 119–263, 337–420; **18**, 9–59, 150–197, 267–303 (facsimile reprint Felinfach: Llanerch Publishers, 1993).

CLA1   Lowe, E.A. 1935 *Codices Latini antiquiores, Part II: Great Britain and Ireland* (1st edn). Oxford. Clarendon Press.

CLA2   Lowe, E.A. 1972 *Codices Latini antiquiores, Part II: Great Britain and Ireland* (2nd edn). Oxford. Clarendon Press.

OSL   *Ordnance Survey Letters, Mayo, vol. 1, 1838.* (MS in Royal Irish Academy.)

PG   Migne, J.P. 1857–66 *Patrologia Graeca,* vols 1–161. Paris. The author.

Full references

Alexander, J.J.G. 1978 *Insular manuscripts from the 6th to the 9th century.* London. Harvey Miller.

Anderson, A.O. and Anderson, M.O. 1961 *Adomnan's Life of Columba.* London and Edinburgh. Nelson.

Anderson, M.O. 1991 *Adomnan's Life of Columba.* Oxford. Clarendon Press (revised edn of Anderson and Anderson 1961).

Armstrong, E.C.R. 1916 The Shrine of the Cathach (Appendix I of H.J. Lawlor, The Cathach of St Columba). *Proceedings of the Royal Irish Academy* **33**C (1916–17), 390–6.

Armstrong, E.C.R. and Lawlor, H.J. 1918 *Proceedings of the Royal Irish Academy* **34**, 96–126.

Arnaud-Lindet, M.-P. (ed.) 1990 *Orose, histoires (contre les Païens),* Tome I, Livres I–III. Paris. Les Belles Lettres.

Badawy, Alexander 1978 *Coptic art and archaeology.* Cambridge, Mass. MIT Press.

Best, R.I. and O'Brien, M.A. 1967 *The Book of Leinster.* Dublin. Dublin Institute for Advanced Studies.

Betham, W. 1826 *Irish antiquarian researches,* Part 1. Dublin. William Curry, Jun. and Co., and Hodges and MacArthur.

Bieler, L. 1963 *Ireland, harbinger of the Middle Ages.* London. Oxford University Press.

Bober, H. 1967 On the illumination of the Glazier Codex, a contribution to early Coptic art and its relation to Hiberno-Saxon
interlace. In H. Lehmann-Haupt (ed.), *Homage to a bookman:
essays on manuscripts, books and printing written for Hans P.
Kraus on his 60th birthday, Oct. 12, 1967*, 31–49. Berlin.
Gebr. Mann Verlag.

Breen, A. 1992 The liturgical materials in MS Oxford, Bodleian
Library, Auct. F.4./32. *Archiv für Liturgiewissenschaft* **34**,
121–53.

Campbell, J.L. 1986 *Canna: the story of a Hebridean island*. Oxford.
Oxford University Press.

Carney, J. 1964 *The poems of Blathmac*. London. Irish Texts Society.

Clancy, T.O. and Márkus, G. 1995 *Iona: the earliest poetry of a Celtic
monastery*. Edinburgh. Edinburgh University Press.

Colgan, J. 1647 *Triadis thaumaturgae seu divorum Patricii, Columbae
et Brigida…Acta*. Louvain. Cornelius Coenestenius.

Cuppage, J. *et al.* 1986 *Archaeological survey of the Dingle Peninsula.
Suirbhé seandálaíochta Chorca Dhuibhne*. Ballyferriter.
Oidhreacht Chorca Dhuibhne.

Dinneen. P. (ed.) 1908 *The history of Ireland by Geoffrey Keating,
D.D.* London. Irish Texts Society.

Duignan, L. 1973 A hand-pin from Treanmacmurtagh Bog, Co. Sligo.
Journal of the Royal Society of Antiquaries of Ireland **103**,
220–23.

Duval, P.-M. 1977 *Les Celtes*. Lyons. Gallimard.

Dyer, J. 1989 Monastic psalmody of the Middle Ages. *Revue
Benedictine* **99**, 41–74.

Fischer, B. 1952 Die Lesungen der römischen Ostervigil unter Gregor
dem Großen. In B. Fischer and V. Fiala (eds), *Colligere
fragmenta: Festschrift für Alban Dold*, 144–59. Beuren in
Hohenzollern. Erzabtei Beuren.

Fulford, M.G. 1989 Byzantium and Britain: a Mediterranean
perspective of post-Roman Mediterranean imports in western
Britain and Ireland. *Medieval Archaeology* **33**, 1–6.

Gillespie, F. 1995 Gaelic families of County Donegal. In W. Nolan, L.
Ronayne and M. Dunlevy (eds), *Donegal history and society*,
759–838. Templeogue. Geography Publications.

Haseloff, G. 1990 *Email im frühen Mittelalter*. Marburg. Hitzeroth.

Hayes, R. 1949 *Biographical dictionary of Irishmen in France*. Dublin.
M.H. Gill.

Heine, R.F. 1995 *Gregory of Nyssa's treatise on the inscriptions of the
Psalms*. Oxford. Clarendon Press.

Henderson, G. 1987 *From Durrow to Kells*. London. Thames and
Hudson.

Hennessy, W.M. and Kelly, D.H. 1875 *The Book of Fenagh*. Dublin.
Alexander Thom.

Henry, F. 1945 Remains of the early Christian period on Inishkea North, Co. Mayo. *Journal of the Royal Society of Antiquaries of Ireland* **75**, 127–55.

Henry, F. 1950 Les débuts de la miniature irlandaise. Gazette des Beaux-Arts **37**, 5–34.

Henry, F. 1951 New monuments from Inishkea North, Co. Mayo. *Journal of the Royal Society of Antiquaries of Ireland* **81**, 65–9.

Henry, F. 1965 *Irish art in the early Christian period (to 800 A.D.).* London. Methuen.

Herbert, M. 1988 *Iona, Kells and Derry: the history and hagiography of the monastic familia of Columba.* Dublin. Four Courts Press (repr. 1996).

Herity, M. 1989 The antiquity of An Turas (The Pilgrimage Round) in Ireland. In A. Lehner and W. Berschin (eds), *Lateinische Kultur im VIII. Jahrhundert,* 95–143. St. Ottilien. E.O.S. Verlag.

Herity, M. 1995a Two island hermitages in the Atlantic: Rathlin O'Birne, Donegal, and Caher Island, Mayo. *Journal of the Royal Society of Antiquaries of Ireland* **125**, 85–128.

Herity, M. 1995b The Chi-Rho and other early cross-forms in Ireland. In J.-M. Picard (ed.), *Aquitaine and Ireland in the Middle Ages,* 233–60. Dublin. Four Courts Press.

Herity, M. 2000 The return of the Cathach to Ireland. In A.P. Smith (ed.), *Seanchas: essays in early medieval archaeology, history and literature in honour of Francis J. Byrne,* 454–64. Dublin. Four Courts Press.

Historical Manuscripts Commission 1902 Calendar of the Stuart Papers. London. HMSO.

Hunt, R.W. 1961 *Saint Dunstan's classbook from Glastonbury: Codex Biblioth. Bodleianae Oxon. Auct. F.4./32.* Amsterdam. North Holland Publishing Company.

Lacey, B. 1998 *Manus O'Donnell: the Life of Colum Cille.* Dublin. Four Courts Press.

Lacy, B. *et al.* 1983 *Archaeological survey of County Donegal.* Lifford. Donegal County Council.

Lapidge, M. 1983 Latin learning in Dark Age Wales: some prolegomena. In D. Ellis Evans (ed.), *Proceedings of the seventh international congress of Celtic studies, held at Oxford, 10–15 July 1983,* 91–107. Oxford. D. Ellis Evans.

Lawlor, H.J. 1916 The Cathach of St Columba. *Proceedings of the Royal Irish Academy* **33** (1916–17), 241–443.

Linton, O. 1961 The interpretation of the Psalms in the early Christian church. *Studia Patristica* **4**, 143–56.

Macalister, R.A.S. 1945 *Corpus inscriptionum insularum Celticarum.* Volume I. Dublin. Stationery Office.

Macalister, R.A.S. 1949 *Corpus inscriptionum insularum Celticarum.* Volume II. Dublin. Stationery Office.

Mc Carthy, Dan 2001 'The chronology of Saint Colum Cille', paper presented at Tionól 2001, 23–4 November 2001, School of Celtic Studies, Dublin Institute for Advanced Studies. The paper was accessed at www.celt.dias.ie/english/tionol/tionol01.html on 14 December 2001.

McDonough, J. 1962 *Gregorii Nysseni: Inscriptiones in Psalmorum; In sextum Psalmum; In Ecclesiasten.* Leiden. Brill.

Mac Niocaill, G. 1990 The Irish 'Charters'. In P. Fox (ed.), *The Book of Kells, MS 58, Trinity College Library, Dublin: commentary*, 153–65. Luzern. Fine Art Facsimile Publishers of Switzerland / Facsimile Verlag.

McNamara, M. 1973 *Psalter text and Psalter study in the early Irish church* (A.D. 600–1200). *Proceedings of the Royal Irish Academy* **73**C, 201–98.

McNamara, M. 1998 Some affiliations of the St Columba series of Psalm headings: a preliminary study (Part 1). *Proceedings of the Irish Biblical Association* **21**, 87–111.

McNamara, M. 1999 Some affiliations of the St Columba series of Psalm headings: a preliminary study (Part 2). *Proceedings of the Irish Biblical Association* **22**. 91–123. (Repr., with Part 1, in 2000 in M. McNamara, *The Psalms in the early Irish Church*. Sheffield. Sheffield Academic Press.)

Nic Dhonnchadha, L. 1964 *Aided Muirchertaigh Meic Erca*. Dublin. Dublin Institute for Advanced Studies.

Nordenfalk, C. 1947 Before the Book of Durrow. *Acta Archaeologica* **18**, 141–74.

Ó Cochláin, R.S. 1968 The Cathach, battle book of the O'Donnells. *The Irish Sword* **8**, 157–77.

O'Curry, E. 1861 *Lectures on the manuscript materials of ancient Irish history*. Dublin. James Duffy.

Ó Floinn, R. 1995 Sandhills, silver and shrines: fine metalwork of the medieval period from Donegal. In W. Nolan, L. Ronayne and M. Dunlevy (eds), *Donegal history and society*, 85–148. Templeogue: Geography Publications.

O'Kelleher, A. and Schoepperle, G. 1918 *Betha Colaim Chille, Life of Columcille. Compiled by Manus O'Donnell in 1532*. Illinois. University of Illinois. (Repr. 1994 by Dublin Institute for Advanced Studies.)

Ó Riain, P. 1985 *Corpus genealogiarum sanctorum Hiberniae*. Dublin. Dublin Institute for Advanced Studies.

Pächt, O. 1986 *Book illumination in the Middle Ages: an introduction*. London. Harvey Miller and Oxford University Press.

Penna, A. 1959 I titoli del Salterio siriaco e S. Gerolamo. *Biblica* **40**, 177–87.

Plummer, Charles 1910 *Vitae sanctorum Hiberniae*. 2 vols. Oxford. Clarendon Press.

Raftery, B. 1983 *A catalogue of Irish Iron Age antiquities*. Marburg. Veröffentlichung des Vorgeschichtlichen Seminars Marburg.

Rahlfs, A. 1979 *Psalmi cum Odis. Septuaginta Vetus Testamentum Graecum X* (3rd edn). Göttingen. Vandenhoeck & Ruprecht.

Ralegh Radford, C.A. 1956 Imported pottery found at Tintagel, Cornwall. In D.B. Harden (ed.) *Dark-Age Britain*, 59–70. London. Methuen.

Reeves, W. 1857 *The Life of St Columba*. Dublin. The Irish Archaeological and Celtic Society.

Richardson, H. 1987 Observations on Christian art in early Ireland, Georgia and Armenia. In M. Ryan (ed.), *Ireland and insular Art, AD 500–1200*, 129–37. Dublin. Royal Irish Academy (repr. 2002).

Rondeau, M.-J. 1958 Une nouvelle preuve de l'influence d'Eusèbe de Césarée sur Athanase: l'interprétation des Psaumes. *Recherches de Science Religieuse* **56**, 385–434.

Roth, U. 1979 Studien zur Ornamentik frühchristlicher Handschriften des insularen Bereichs von den Anfängen bis zum Book of Durrow. *Bericht der Römisch-Germanischen Kommission* **60**, 7–225.

Salmon, Pierre 1959 *Les 'Tituli Psalmorum' des manuscrits latins (Collectanea Biblica Latina XII)*. Rome. Vatican.

Salmon, Pierre 1962 *The breviary through the centuries*. Collegeville, Minnesota. Liturgical Press.

Schauman, B.T. 1978 The Irish script of the MS Milan, Biblioteca Ambrosiana, S. 45 sup. (ante ca. 625). *Scriptorium* **32**, 3–18.

Sharpe, R. 1995 *Adomnán of Iona: Life of St Columba*. Harmondsworth. Penguin.

Smyth, A.P. 1984 *Warlords and holy men, Scotland AD 80–1000*. London. Edward Arnold.

Thomas, A.C. 1959 Imported pottery in Dark Age western Britain. *Medieval Archaeology* **3**, 89–111.

Thomas, A.C. 1981 *A provisional list of imported pottery in post-Roman western Britain and Ireland*. Redruth. Institute of Cornish Studies.

Vian, G.M. 1991 Il *De Psalmorum titulis*: il esegesi di Attanasio tra Eusebio e Cirillo. *Orpheus* **12**, 93–132.

Wilde, W.R. 1861 *A descriptive catalogue of the antiquities of animal materials and bronze in the museum of the Royal Irish Academy*. Dublin. Hodges, Smith and Co.

Wilde, W.R. 1867 *Lough Corrib, its shores and islands*. Dublin. McGlashan and Gill.

Williams, N.J.A. 1980 *Poems of Giolla Brighde mac Con Midhe*. London. Irish Texts Society.

Woolfenden, G.W. 1993 The use of the Psalter by early monastic communities. *Studia Patristica* **26**, 88–94.

Appendix 1

Irish placenames mentioned in the *Cathach* booklet, pp 1–60

Placename	*County*
Armagh	Armagh
Assaroe	Donegal
Ballymagrorty	Donegal
Ballyshannon	Donegal
Bealach Buidhe	Roscommon
Bangor	Down
Boyle	Roscommon
Caher Island	Mayo
Clonamery	Kilkenny
Clonmacnoise	Offaly
Cong	Mayo
Conwal	Donegal
Cúl Drebene (Cooldrumman)	Sligo
Derry	Londonderry
Devenish Island	Fermanagh
Dromsnat	Monaghan
Drumcliff	Sligo
Drumhome	Donegal
Dulane	Meath
Durrow	Offaly
Elphin	Roscommon
Fearsad Mór	Donegal
Fenagh	Leitrim
Gartan	Donegal
Glasnevin	Dublin
Glend Colaim Cilli (Gleann Choluim Cille / Glencolmcille)	Donegal
Glendalough	Wicklow
Illauntannig	Kerry
Inishkea Islands	Mayo
Kells	Meath
Killeen	Mayo
Kilmacrenan	Donegal
Kilmore	Cavan
Kilshannig	Kerry
Kilvickadownig	Kerry

Knockane	Kerry
Lambay	Dublin
Letterkenny	Donegal
Lifford	Donegal
Loch Beagh	Donegal
Maumanorig	Kerry
Moone	Kildare
Moville	Down
Moylurg	Roscommon
Nendrum	Down
Newport	Mayo
Racoon	Donegal
Ramelton	Donegal
Rathlin O'Birne Island	Donegal
Swords	Dublin
Tara	Meath
Treanmacmurtagh Bog	Sligo

Appendix 2

Pages 7–10 (reproduction at 60% of original) of 'Report on the repair and rebinding of the *Cathach* together with further notes and observations' by Roger Powell († 1990)

It is clear that Lawlor was not conversant with the practice of Irish and other Insular scribes in preparing vellum leaves for writing. What follows is put forward in the light of experience in dealing with many Insular manuscript books from Trinity College, Dublin, The Royal Irish Academy and elsewhere including The Book of Durrow, The Book of Armagh, The Lichfield St. Chad Gospels, A.II.27 from Durham, The Book of Kells and in examining The Stonyhurst Gospel of St. John for "The Relics of St. Cuthbert", Durham Cathedral and "The Stonyhurst Gospel of St. John", the Roxburghe Club.

In attempting to establish the original quiring of The Cathach of St. Columba the starting point is the tendency for Irish and Irish-inspired mss. to be arranged in 10-leaf quires, usually of 5 conjoint bifolia. Applying this to The Cathach, on ff.9, 19, 29, 39 and 49 the pricking for ruling (meticulously on the vertical rules) and especially the ruling (meticulously confined within the vertical rules) is markedly heavier than on the following nine leaves where it gradually fades away. This shows that both pricking and ruling was performed from the top leaf of each assembled quire and that there was no re-ruling of the lower leaves. That there is now no trace of ruling on the lower leaves does not mean that there were no impressions when it was ruled; the damp conditions over hundreds of years and the immersion by Betham when separating the leaves allowed recovery. The fact that re-ruling was not always necessary, though often practised in later ms., is an interesting comment on the different character of early vellum compared with what is available today.

Comparing the hair and flesh sides of the quiring suggested

by the pricking and ruling from f.9 to the end shows that except for single leaves at ff.10 and 17 and ff.21 and 26 the remainder was made up of 23 conjoint bifolia, so confirming the 10-leaf quiring, and in turn suggesting that ff.1 - 8 are what remains of a 10-leaf quire of which the first two leaves (now missing) were conjoint with ff.8 and 7 and having hair-sides on verso and recto respectively. Within the quire the arrangement of hair and flesh sides is indiscrimminate with a slight tendency for flesh-sides to be outwards.

There is some evidence that while the ms. was in single leaves it was stabbed (in quires?), perhaps with a thread passing through one, two and possibly three widely separated holes. These holes appear in or near the inner margins near the head and equi-distant from head and tail. The middle one is clearly vissible from f.3 - f.28. One near the head is visible from f.8 - f.28. Two further series only visible at the head seem to run from f.29 - f.38 and from f.39 - f.48.

An area of pricked(?) holes in the middle of f.58 penetrates decreasingly through the preceding leaves; one, undoubtedly a piercing, persists through to f.32.

Roger Powell.

Key for diagram overleaf:-

⦂	Red dots in manuscript, recto or verso indicated.
▧	Other colour on initials, recto or verso indicated.
△	Small hole pierced half-way up inner edge of folio.
☉	Folio pierced at inner head, green stain begins the run.
☐	Folio pierced at centre, green stain.
⓺	Folio pierced at centre head, rusty stain.
⊛	Folio pierced over central area up to fifteen times.

PROBABLE GATHERINGS	HAIR SIDE				
Folio 1	R	Reversed in replacement.			
2	R	Folio 3 previously, reversed in replacement.			
3	R	Folio 2 previously, reversed in replacement.			△
4	V				△
5	V				△
6	V				△
7	V		○V		△
8	R		○V		△
9	V			◎	△
10	R			◎	△
11	V		○RV	◎	△
12	R	Reversed in replacement.	☑V	◎	△
13	V			◎	△
14	R		○RV ☑RV	◎	△
15	V		○V ☑V	◎	△
16	R			◎	△
17	R		○V ☑V	◎	△
18	R		○V ☑V	◎	△
19	V		○R ☑R	◎	△
20	V		○V	◎	△
21	V		○RV ☑RV	◎	△
22	V		○V ☑R	◎	△
23	V		○RV ☑RV	◎	△
24	R		○V	◎	△
25	R		○R ☑R	◎	△
26	V			◎	△
27	R			◎	△
28	R		○V	◎	

PROBABLE GATHERINGS	HAIR SIDE					
Folio 29	V				⊘	
30	V		◌V	☑V	⊘	
31	V		◌V	☑V	⊘	
32	V		◌V	☑V	⊘	
33	V		◌V		⊘	
34	R		◌V	☑V	⊘	⊡
35	R	Folio 36 previously.	◌RV	☑V	⊘	⊡
36	R	Folio 35 previously.	◌V	☑V	⊘	⊡
37	R				⊘	⊡
38	R				⊘	⊡
39	R		◌V	☑V		⊡
40	V		◌R	☑R		⊡
41	V		◌RV	☑RV		⊡
42	V	Folio 43 previously.				⊡
43	R	Folio 42 previously.		☑V	⊚	⊡
44	V			☑V	⊘ ⊚	⊡
45	R				⊘ ⊚	⊡
46	R				⊘ ⊚	⊡
47	R				⊘ ⊚	⊡
48	V				⊘ ⊚	⊡
49	R				⊘ ⊚	⊡
50	V				⊘ ⊚	⊡
51	V				⊘ ⊚	⊡
52	V				⊘ ⊚	⊡
53	R				⊘	⊡
54	V				⊘	⊡
55	R				⊘	⊡
56	R				⊘	⊡
57	R				⊘	⊡
58	V				⊘	⊡

Appendix 3
The Springmount Bog wax tablets

The following is an extract from a paper by Martin McNamara on 'Psalter text and psalter study in the early Irish Church (AD 600–1200), published in *Proceedings of the Royal Irish Academy* 73C (1973), 201–98, and updated by Fr McNamara in 2001–2002 for this publication. It also includes extracts from the late Dr Maurice Sheehy's Appendix to the above paper, pp 277–80, and his reading of the text on fol. 3v of the tablets.

These tablets were found in Springmount Bog, about half a mile from the village of Clough, Co. Antrim, and seven miles north of Ballymena. They were purchased by the National Museum of Ireland in 1914 from Mr W. Gregg of Clough. The tablets probably come from an ancient monastery.

They consist of a book of six wooden 'leaves', inlaid with wax on both sides of each (except the two outer ones, which have no wax on the outside). The six tablets when found were bound together as a book by a thong of leather stitching which passed through the holes perforating one edge of the tablets, thus forming a loose spine; two bands of leather were placed around the book, at the top and the bottom. The tablets measure approximately 21cm by 7.7cm and each is 6 to 7mm thick.

The tablets contain the text of Psalms 30–32 (in the Vulgate numbering). The text is Gallican, with some readings due to the influence of the Old Latin and others arising, it would appear, from carelessness in transcription or from the fact that the writer depended on his memory.

The tablets were probably used in primary instruction, to initiate a pupil into the arts of reading and writing through the psalter, or Book of Psalms, as was the custom. The scribe in this instance was probably the schoolmaster. The purpose of the tablets probably explains the inaccuracies of transcription.

The original editors, Armstrong and Macalister (1920) made no attempt to date the tablets. Dr Bernhard Bischoff, in a letter to J.N. Hillgarth (Hillgarth 1962, 183), noted that the script of the tablets has the same cursive characteristics as the fragments of Isidore in MS St. Gall 1399 a. 1 (seventh century) and Codex Usserianus Primus (Trinity College, Dublin, 55; beginning of seventh century), both of which are in Irish script. The tablets would thus be of a seventh-century date. In a more detailed study, D.H. Wright (1963) dates them to about AD 600.

Since Wright's contribution, studies on the palaeography of the tablets have been made by B. Schauman (1974, 308–10; 1979, 35–7) in particular but also by T. Julian Brown (1982, 104; 1984, 312, 320, 321) and W. O'Sullivan (1994, 177–9). With regard to the date to be assigned to them, Bischoff (1990, 14 n. 43), with reference to Wright (1963, 219), says that they may be dated around AD 600. According to Schauman (1979, 37) the archaic features of the script argue against a date as late as the seventh century and in favour of a rather early date for the tablets. In her opinion it is not unreasonable to place them in the sixth century; indeed, she believes they may well represent a type of hand common in Ireland as early as St Patrick's day. In T. Julian Brown's (1982, 104) opinion the tablets cannot be dated by internal evidence, and it is perhaps enough to ascribe them to the first half of the seventh century. David Dumville (1999, 31–5) reviews the various opinions put forward with regard to the script and date of the tablets. Despite Bischoff's rejection of the likelihood of an import from Bobbio (Bischoff in Hillgarth 1962, 183 n. 78), Dumville (1999, 35) remarks that while it might seem simpler to rule any scribe from abroad out of consideration, it is not absolutely to be excluded that these tablets were written in the context of sixth- (or fifth-) century British missionary endeavour in Ireland.

Despite this observation, the almost unanimous scholarly opinion is that in these tablets we have one of the oldest extant specimens of Irish writing. The tablets also provide precious evidence that even at this early date pupils were being initiated into the arts of reading and writing through the Gallican text of the psalter, not through the Old Latin. And, in fact, it is the Gallican text, and it alone, that we shall find as the biblical text used in all later Irish commentaries.

Folio 3v of the tablets (below) represents Psalm 31:1–7a. <Angle brackets> indicate missing or illegible text, [square brackets] indicate editorial emendation.

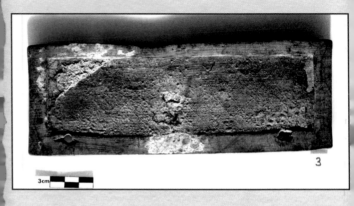

Folio 3v of the Springmount Bog wax tablets. (© National Museum of Ireland

Column 1
<Beati, quoru>m remisse sunt iniquitates
<et quoru>m tecta sunt peccata.
<Beat>us vir cui non inpotavit Dominus peccatum,
<n>ec est in spiritu eius dolos. Quoniam t<a>cui in-
<ve>teraverunt in me ossa mea d<um cla>ma-
rem tota die. Quoniam die ac nocte
gravata est super me m<anu>s t<u>a,
conversus sum in er<?>omna mea,
dum configitur mihi spina.

Column 2
Dilictum meum cognitum tibi fe<ci>
et iniustiam meam non absco<ndi>.
Dixi: confitebor adversus me [iniustitiam meam Domino] et <tu>
rimisisti impietatem peccati mei.
Pro hac orabit ad te omnis sanctis in
tempore oportuno,
verumtamen in diluvio aquarum
multarum ad [eu]m non proximabunt.
Tu es refugium meum